A guide to precision reflexology

To Andrew, Ben, John and Patrick

An old Japanese foot tale

Otau was a wise, old and wrinkled man. The whole village respected his healing abilities.

One day a foreigner came to ask him many questions and write down the healing ways of Otau.

However, all Otau would say was, 'See to their feet and you have seen to their body.'

'I do not understand,' insisted the foreigner.

'Your understanding will never be enough,' Otau chuckled. 'See to their feet and that will be enough.'

A guide to precision reflexology

by
Jan Williamson

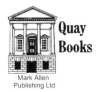

Quay Books

Mark Allen
Publishing Ltd

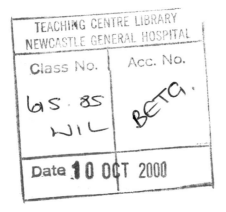
Quay Books Division, Mark Allen Publishing Ltd, Jesses Farm, Dinton, Nr Salisbury, Wiltshire, SP3 5HN

British Library Cataloguing-in-Publication Data
A catalogue record is available for this book

© Mark Allen Publishing Ltd 1999
ISBN 1 85642 176 7

Printed in the United Kingdom by Redwood Books, Trowbridge, Wiltshire

Contents

Acknowledgements

My deepest thanks to:

* Prue for her trust and great generosity and to,
* Stewart for the inspiration and for his confidence in me.

Thank you to Sue, Val and Sally for the photographs and to John J Williamson for his artwork. The reflexology charts in this book are produced by kind courtesy of Prue Miskin.

Preface

The aim of this book is to introduce a specific style of reflexology, to explain how and when it can be given and to establish its position within the field of complementary therapies. Hopefully, I will also share my enthusiasm for a therapy which I have found, within clinical practice, to be extremely effective. Perhaps then it is also no coincidence that it is enjoyable both to give and to receive.

Reflexology, along with other therapies, is constantly developing and growing, as is my approach to it. This book represents my perceptions at this time. There are many valid and effective approaches to reflexology, precision reflexology being one of them. This is not a definitive guide but, rather, just one step along the way.

There is, within the world of reflexology, a constant debate about the variety of different charts or 'maps' used. To put this into perspective we need to be aware that when reflexology originated, 5000 years ago in the East, there was no need for a chart, each treatment being a response between the practitioner's sensitivity and intuition and the recipient's energy levels. This should be the underlying principle behind treatment today. The reality of the reflexes is in the practitioner's fingers. The charts are a Western influence, they are necessary as a guide to student learning — but they are simply that, a guide. Given time, students develop and learn to trust their own sensitivity.

Precision reflexology requires therapists to develop their sense of touch, connecting with the client on an energetic level and responding appropriately, aiming to restore a natural equilibrium.

Foreword

I would first like to say how delighted I am that this excellently clear and much needed book has been written. 'How did the linking start?' you might ask. Well, I had been practising various mind, body and energy therapies for many years before I discovered reflexology in 1975 and found it to be the best of them all, combining all the qualities I most valued; a wide range of availability, good for self-help and effective on so many levels. So I ran a practice for a while and later ran a school for twelve years. During this time I was finding some of the body work techniques worked well on the feet, with exciting results.

Jan Williamson joined me five years ago and we ran the school together, developing the linking with the help of our students. Now I have happily retired and Jan runs the school herself. We now both run short postgraduate courses where we are being constantly asked for a book on linking and precision reflexology and, here it is.

The method has proved so popular that Jan has formed the Federation of Precision Reflexologists. There is a referral register for those who have experienced the benefits to find others practising this method in other areas of the country.

I think that one reason for its popularity is that it is an exciting addition to whatever technique is being used and will enhance and energise your treatments. The results will quickly make sense of any extra time spent. It also encourages the worker to tune into and use their client's energy whenever possible, it develops our receptive qualities and makes for accuracy.

The linking between organs, glands and the various systems, with no two clients quite the same, is an enlivening challenge and will open doors for you all. It can allow you to pleasurably develop your own creative and holistic thinking. So never a dull moment from now on.

Finally, a big thank you to Jan and my best wishes to you all, enjoy your linking, your surprising results and happy clients.

Prue Miskin
November, 1988

1
Reflexology

While the practice of reflexology is a relatively recent development in the field of complementary therapy in the Western world, it is an ancient holistic healing technique derived from oriental philosophy. This philosophy regards the human being as a miniature version of the universe. Man forms an organic part of nature and is clearly linked to nature. The terminology used by reflexologists such as balance, harmony and energy do not translate easily into Western physiological understanding.

Reflexology is based on the premise that energy channels run throughout the body. The efficacy of the therapy is believed to be the result of stimulation of this energy flow. It is essential to have a basic understanding of this phenomenon. The Indian Yogis call it 'prana', the Chinese call it 'chi', in the West homoeopaths have called it 'vital energy' and 'life force'. Reflexology deals with this internal energy and accepts that the body is a dynamic energy system which is constantly changing.

Oriental belief is that all life is linked to natural rhythms and laws of the universe.The health of each individual depends on a balance in the natural world, while the health of each organ depends on its relationship to all other organs. Nothing can change without changing the whole. Humans are directly and indirectly affected by the cosmic forces which are beyond our control. The optimum state is that each individual should live in harmony with nature and the environment. The aim of reflexology, along with other holistic therapies, is to connect to a person's energy system, to adjust it and harmonise it with the world in which that person lives.

All life can be said to be an expression of energy. In human beings this shows itself in various forms — spiritual, emotional, mental and physical. These are all one and the same energy. Holistic therapies acknowledge that imbalances in one level of energy affect other levels and they aim to restore balance within the entire system.

As an holistic healing technique (the term holistic is from the Greek word 'holos' which means whole), reflexology treats each individual as an entity of body, mind and spirit. It does not treat symptomatically and does not work on a specific system in a technical manner but, rather, it works with the whole person. The aim being to restore the individual into a state of balance. Because the nature of the whole is always different from the mere sum of its parts, the whole system cannot be properly understood by studying individual parts. It is vital to see each person as an integrated organisation.

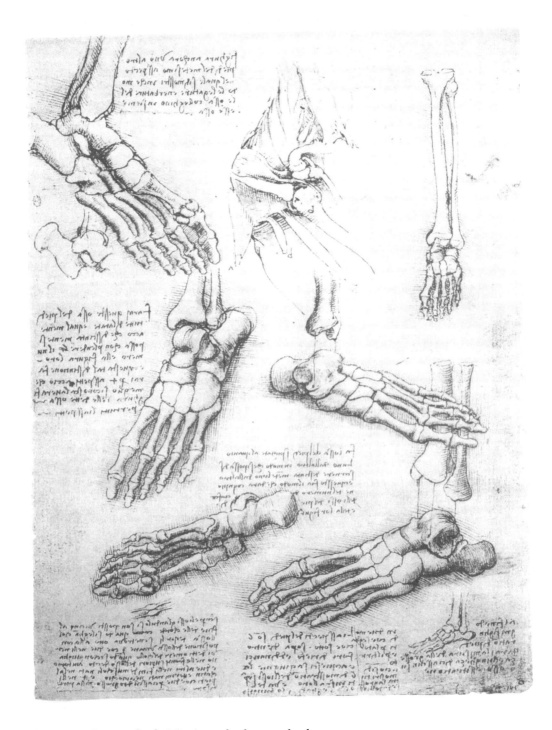

Figure 1.1: Leonardo da Vinci on the human body

Reflexology opens up energy channels in the body. Specific techniques are used to apply pressure to the feet which create channels for energy to circulate throughout the body.

History

Leonardo da Vinci (1452–1519) said that the feet are 'a masterpiece of engineering and a work of art' (see *Figure 1.1*). The feet certainly have a special place and a fascination in mythology, religion and culture over the centuries. In mythology the famous reference is that of Achilles' heel, meaning a vulnerable area. The removal of shoes at the threshold of holy places for the Buddhists, the Hindus and the Muslims is compulsory. The North American Indians also regard the feet with high esteem. A Cherokee, Jenny Wallace, says,

> *'The feet walk upon the earth and through this your spirit is connected to the universe. Our feet are our contact with the earth and the energies that flow through it'.*

Among reflexologists it is a widely held theory that reflexology originated in China some 5000 years ago, and there is Egyptian documentation dating from around 2500–2300 BC. In the tomb of Ankhmahor, a highly respected physician, there are wall paintings showing what appears to be the practice of reflexology (see *Figure 1.2*). The inscription below this scene reads, *'Do not let it be painful'* says a patient and the attendant replies *'I do as you please'*. The origins of reflexology are in ancient history when pressure therapies were recognised and accepted as preventative and therapeutic.

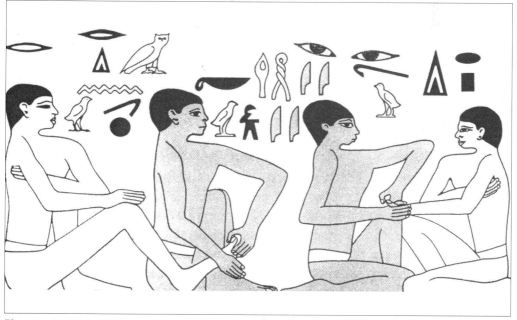

Figure 1.2

The art of reflexology was also known 500 years ago in India. In an Hindu painting of the god Vishnu, the feet symbolise the unity of the entire universe (see *Figure 1.3*). In the same way that Eastern philosophies see the individual being as a microcosm of the universe, so the feet represent the energy of the body.

There is also documentation, dated from the 2nd century BC, describing a Chinese doctor Yu Fu (meaning foot healing) who healed patients with massage.

The earliest records of the European influence on reflexology appear to be in 1582, when Dr Adamus and Dr A'tatis wrote a book on zone therapy. This describes the feet divided into longitudinal zones, with corresponding areas on the body. Western, scientific studies into the neurological function of the body can be traced to Sir Henry Head working in London in the 1890s. He studied the sensory pathways of the body and, with a fellow physician, WHR Rivers, he proved the neurological connection between the skin and the internal organs.

At the same time, in Germany Dr Alfons Cornelius was working on the fact that pressure points operate within nerve pathways and produce a reaction in a distant part of the body. In 1902, he published a book 'Druckpunkte, or pressure points, their origin and significance'.

The American influence came with Dr William Fitzgerald (1872–1942) who 'discovered' reflexology while travelling in Vienna at the turn of the century. He was able to show that pressure applied to one area on a foot anaesthetised a corresponding area of the body. This led him to use reflexology in the management of pain. He co-authored a book with a colleague, Dr Edwin Bowers, in 1917 entitled 'Zone therapy'. This work was further developed by Dr Joe Shelby Riley who devised a 'hooking technique' to apply specific pressure. He made the first detailed diagrams of the reflex areas located on the feet. A therapist, Eunice Ingham, worked with Dr Riley in America in the 1930s. She made a significant contribution to reflexology with detailed 'maps' of the reflex areas of the feet and she wrote two books 'Stories the Feet can tell' and 'Stories the Feet have told'. In these she explains that, because feet are so responsive to touch, it is possible that by applying pressure to the various reflexology points on the feet, a definite therapeutic effect can be produced which is far beyond mere pain control.

Sir Charles Sherrington (1861–1952) conducted experiments with the reflex action and coined the term proprioception — meaning how the body's nervous and muscular systems are co-ordinated together. He proved that the entire nervous system responds to an external stimulus. At its most reduced level reflexology could be described as an 'external stimulus'. In 1932, Sherrington was awarded the Nobel prize for his work.

Doreen Bayly, a student of Eunice Ingham, introduced reflexology into Britain in the 1960s. Since then it has become increasingly popular and it is now recognised as a valid form of complementary care. A survey conducted by Professor Ernst of Exeter University in 1996 showed that 32% of those surveyed had received reflexology.

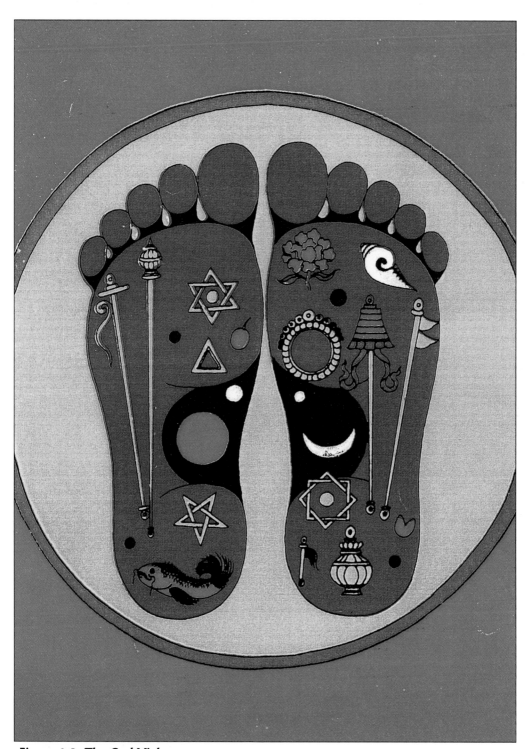

Figure 1.3: The God Vishnu

Rationale

Reflexologists believe that the feet represent the energy of the body. For example, it is believed that the big toe corresponds to the the head (see *Figure 1.4*).

The reflex area for the spine is located on the medial aspect of each foot. The reflex areas for the organs and structures of the right side of the body are on the right foot and those of the left side are on the left foot (see *Figure 1.5*).

Reflex areas are on both dorsal and plantar aspects of the feet. The same principles apply to the hands (see *Figure 1.6*).

There are many rationales put forward for reflexology. They reflect its history through Eastern and Western societies. They may refer to the Western influence regarding the neurological and circulatory systems, for example, Doreen Bayly believes that there is an electrical type impulse triggered off by pressure massage on a tender reflex point that can produce a subtle flow of energy, bringing a return of vitality to each person during treatment. Also, Eunice Ingham said that the nerves of the body can be likened to an electrical system and that reflexology releases tension in that system.

The Eastern approach revolves around concepts of subtle energy, with reference to chakras and meridians. The aim is to restore the natural equilibrium that the body strives to attain.

We also cannot underestimate the value of receiving undivided care and attention and of promoting deep relaxation, thus providing an optimum situation for the restoration of health.

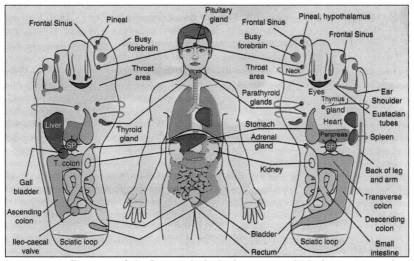

Figure 1.4: Reflex areas of the feet, with the body parts to which they correspond

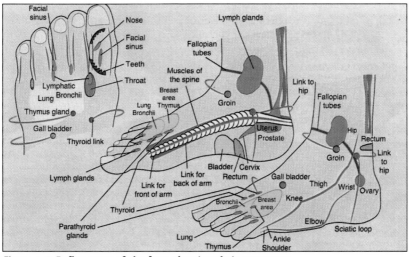

Figure 1.5: Reflex areas of the feet, showing their symmetry

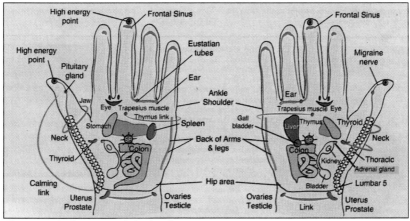

Figure 1.6: Reflex areas of the hands

Application

The reflexology charts are necessary to provide guidance and structure but, rather than being used to deal with one particular symptom, reflexology is used to balance the body's natural equilibrium so that restoration and repair can take place. The Eastern therapeutic approach is that any disease is a result of imbalance, so this therapy is one way to restore that balance and strengthen internal energy.

A thorough knowledge of the location of the reflex areas, of the anatomy and physiology of the body and of the holistic approach to health is required. Practitioners are trained to respond to each treatment with a variety of specific thumb and finger techniques, and to develop sensitivity, so that each consultation is conducted in a caring and responsible manner.

Reflexology can have a positive effect in its ability to relieve stress and tension, whether it be physical or emotional. This often produces an improvement in quality of life. The process of reflexology is not comparable with (diagnostic) methods used in allopathic medicine. Rather, reflexology can be seen as a form of examination which can contribute to an understanding of a condition.

The treatment

As pressure is applied to different reflex points on the feet, different sensations will be felt. A patient's reactions can range from a sharp sensation, to a dull feeling, to a pleasant awareness of pressure. Each treatment is a response to each individual at that time; therefore reactions differ from one person to another and from one treatment to another. One person might experience deep relaxation and another may feel energised. Reflexology is one way, among many, of giving people time to themselves; time to reflect, to relax, to understand their illness and to find some meaning behind it. Rather than suppressing the symptoms, the ethos is to work with the body, both emotionally and physically and to progress accordingly.

Research

There is very little recorded research in reflexology. In 1990, a randomised controlled trial performed by Lafuente *et al* used reflexology in the treatment of headaches. It was a small study, with thirty-two patients randomised to receive drug treatment or reflexology. The study lasted for three months and the results show that improvements were greater in the reflexology group than in the drug group.

In another study in 1992, Petersen *et al* examined reflexology in the treatment of asthma. Thirty patients with bronchial asthma were subdivided at random into two groups. One group received ten weekly reflexology treatments and the other had uniform clinical care. A decrease in consumption of medication and an increase in peak flow levels were observed in the group that received reflexology.

In 1994, Oleson and Flocco used reflexology in the treatment of premenstrual symptoms. This study produced positive results, with a 45% decrease in PMS for the reflexology group, with a 20% decrease in a placebo group. The Department of Complementary Medicine at Exeter University is currently conducting a study to investigate the effects of reflexology on menopausal symptoms.

Anecdotal evidence is now no longer sufficient; all complementary therapies deserve high quality research studies. It is possible to conduct this level of study and still remain true to the principles behind complementary care. In this way, solid evidence can be presented to all healthcare professionals. More importantly, it will enable clients/ patients to make informed choices about their own health management.

Reflexology has ancient foundations and has evolved into the modern world. It has a rationale which is Eastern in philosophy and Western in application. It has become increasingly chosen as a way of improving and maintaining health in a natural way. Although a popular therapy, it is not claimed to be a magical panacea for all ills but most recipients are able to report some degree of improvement in that it helps to alleviate symptoms or reduces their severity. Patients commonly express feelings of improved well-being. The majority of patients find that treatment reduces stress-related disorders, thus helping them to cope better with the pressures of everyday life.

References

Bayly DE (1978) *Reflexology Today*. Thorsons, Wellingborough: 13–14

Centralised Information Service for Complementary Medicine. RCCM (Research Council for Complementary Medicine), Great Ormond Street, London

Dougans I, Ellis S (1992) *The Art of Reflexology*. Element Books, Shaftesbury: 10

Gillanders A (1987) *The Ancient Answer to Modern Ailments*. Ann Gillanders, Harlow: 25–28

Ingham E (1984) *Stories the Feet Have Told*. Ingham Publishing Inc, Saint Petersburg, Florida: 2

Issel C (1990). *Reflexology, Art, Science and History*. New Frontier, Sacramento, California: 172

Oleson T, Flocco W (1993) Randomised controlled study of premenstrual symptoms treated with ear, hand and foot reflexology. *Obs Gynaecol* **82**(6): 906–11

2
Precision reflexology

Precision reflexology is one form of reflexology and, as such, it holds the same rationale as other forms of the therapy. It focuses on stimulating 'reflex points' on the feet in order to maintain good health. Practitioners believe that, by applying appropriate pressure to these points, it is possible to treat a wide range of disorders. Precision reflexology has been developed by Prue Miskin (founder and principal of The School of Precision Reflexology). There is a full practitioner training course based on the charts, ideas and style involved with the precision technique. But also, the primary technique, ie. 'linking' can be adapted to other forms of reflexology.

In order to understand the fundamental principle behind this therapy, it is essential to have an understanding of the origins of all reflexology and, also, of the subtle energy of the body, as explained in *Chapter 1*. The aim of precision reflexology is to connect to a person's energy system, to adjust it and to harmonise it within itself and with the world surrounding that person. Practitioners work with this internal energy and accept that the body is a dynamic energy system which is constantly changing.

Precision work helps the practitioner to understand the client on all levels. It attempts to make sense of the internal 'dialogue' existing within each person. The body has its own multi-directional network of communication. This is not a mechanical process but functions with information and intelligence: it is a form of communication without words.

One important aspect of the unique nature of this technique is that it does not rely on force or actual physical pressure but, rather, it is presented with an element of choice. Each individual client can receive the benefits in a way that is appropriate to him/her at that time. Each person's own energies are used to heal him/herself. It will be appropriate on all levels of their being — physical, mental, emotional and spiritual — all these being one and the same energy. Bearing this approach in mind, it is obvious that the practitioner must be clear about his or her own intention within the treatment; he/she is not imposing his/her will on the client but simply presenting the opportunity for the body to heal itself, using its own innate intelligence. This must be allowed to happen in its own way and in its own time. This process of change is not a conscious decision.

An overall guideline throughout is that of acknowledging a condition or presenting symptom and not opposing or denying it. 'Success' within the treatment situation is often difficult to define in that although it may not necessarily mean a lessening or elimination of the original symptom, it can be shown by less obvious, but perhaps more valuable, signs, that the client feels that the quality of his/her life has improved, or maybe feels more in control of various aspects of that life. Sometimes a positive outcome can be when the recipient of the treatment accepts the symptom as a part of him/herself and 'uses' it, asking questions such as, 'how does this make me feel?' 'why this particular thing at this time?' or 'what does this mean for me?'. This approach obviously is quite different from the standard one of Western medicine.

There is a richness to a positive treatment that is difficult to explain; there is no one single formula, each session being a unique response. There are several necessary elements that could be considered:

1. The skill of the practitioner involving technical knowledge and the ability to respond appropriately to reactions felt during the treatment.

2. The energetic overall state of health of the client; the level of harmony within him/herself and with the environment.

3. The unique, complex relationship between the client and the practitioner. The client needs to feel secure, respected, cared for and attended to. Ideally, there is an atmosphere of mutual respect and trust. The aim is to create an optimum environment for the recipient to fully engage in the session so that he/she can begin to feel empowered and to take responsibility for his/her own health. This daunting task should be a gradual process, as each person feels ready.

4. The experience of the actual treatment can be enjoyable.

Each of these elements reflects the dynamic nature of a treatment, each one responding to another.

Precision reflexology techniques

There are precision reflexology charts that are used in the training of this technique (see *Chapter 1*). The reflex area for the spine is located on the medial aspect of each foot. Reflex areas are on both dorsal and plantar aspects of both feet. The same principles apply to the hands.

The specific technique which is exclusive to this training is called 'linking'. This involves holding two (sometimes three) identified reflex points at the same time to add power and definition to the treatment. As the link is held, the practitioner pauses and is aware of 'listening' via his/her hands and, in this way, the treatment is matched to the individual with precision. This technique can be adapted to all forms of reflexology and it is currently taught to many students who have qualified in other schools.

'Linking' is initiated by stimulating the reflexes to be connected and feeling the energy between them. Once experienced, this feeling will amplify, especially if both the worker and the client are focused. This can be demonstrated on the hands. Points on the thumb and middle finger of each hand are joined together; these are located in the centre of the finger, about a quarter of an inch down from the tip. This can be felt as a small tingle, a pulse, or a feeling of warmth. There are defined sets of links, each producing particular effects and with their own applications; more can also be developed with intuition. Not all of them are for everyone and, in fact, it would not be appropriate to use all the links within a single consultation. The main benefit is that it provides access to the subtle body energies of each client, giving an added dimension to each session and allowing the practitioner to respond fully to the true needs of each person.

The treatment is a response to the recipient at that particular time, therefore reactions differ from one person to another and from one treatment to another. The effects produced range from energising and uplifting to calming and deeply relaxing, so the 'links' ought to be used to 'match' the needs of the receiver. The treatment reflects the energy levels of the receiver with some people being more receptive than others. It is possible to balance body energy and to make the therapy truly holistic, both to give and to receive. Experienced therapists can use this approach with accuracy and sensitivity. Awareness of the subtle body increases knowledge of all aspects of a person; physical, emotional and spiritual. In this way, precision reflexology remains true to the Eastern origins of the therapy.

As with all work of this nature, practitioners need to pay attention to their own energy levels and to care for themselves with diet, exercise, relaxation and breathing techniques.

Precision work has the potential for great power even with gentle pressure, this being particularly effective on painful reflexes or for very fragile and vulnerable clients. The treatment is given without force and it is always presented with great respect for the client. Each person will receive, and progress through, the course of treatment in a way that is correct for them. When, or indeed, if, they begin to benefit it will be exactly as and when they are ready. This then being a truly holistic therapy.

There are specific sets of links that will be explained in detail in the following chapters. Here are some general points to bear in mind which apply to all of them:

- The links need to be held while the practitioner 'listens' responding to the energy of the client. The time to hold will be determined by the needs at that time. After the required time, the worker and, sometimes, the receiver will feel the response diminish. In this way, the technique is self-regulating, the body taking what it requires.
- An extremely energetic link on a person who presents in a sluggish, lethargic manner could indicate an imbalance. However, on a lively, enthusiastic person the same response would be regarded as normal. In the same way, a dull link on a stressed person could be seen as an imbalance and, on a placid, quiet person this would be quite acceptable.

- Each link has its own characteristics, producing its own responses. Clients have a variety of words to describe how they feel, such as, 'relaxed', 'warm', 'floaty', 'lively', 'detached', 'energised' and many more. Some of the links can promote feelings of being expansive and free, others of being deeply relaxed. Some can promote emotional release if the client is ready. The technique is received differently by each person, some feeling the responses isolated to the feet, others feeling reactions in the relevant areas of the body. Practitioners make no judgement about this; it is simply how that person is functioning at the time. If a response is felt in the body, clients use words such as 'glow', 'heat' and 'tingle' to describe how this feels.

- Linking can promote deep relaxation, with the client feeling detached from themselves in a physical sense. It emphasises all the benefits of reflexology and can be applied to a wide range of ailments, some physical and others emotional. All complementary health practitioners are aware of how emotional tension, after a shock, trauma or bereavement, for instance, can become locked into the physical body. There are specific links which can, if the receiver is ready, help to release this pain. Sometimes this is dramatic with a strong emotional response, sometimes it is calm as the client relates a particular incident from their past.

Reflexology has ancient foundations and has evolved into the modern world. Precision reflexology enables practitioners to remain true to the origins, both in the philosophy behind the treatment and in the approach.

References

Pert CB (1998) *Pert Molecules of Emotion*. Simon and Schuster, USA

Cormack M, Mitchell A (1998) *The Therapeutic Relationship in Complementary Health Care*. Churchill Livingstone, Edinburgh

Mitchell S (1998) *Naturopathy*. Element Books, Shaftesbury

3
Balance and harmony

Precision reflexology provides a focus for energy work. The Hindu Chakra system (centres of energy) is one way of explaining this concept (see *Figure 3.1*). Chakras do not exist in a physical sense but they give us a way of defining a difficult concept. In a similar way, the Western way of describing a block of energy is to talk about having 'a lump in the throat' or 'butterflies in the stomach'. Each chakra has many characteristics, including physical, emotional and spiritual qualities; these qualities are all one and the same energy which cannot be separated. This energy can be seen as a way of representing the individual within each of us. The relevance to the 'linking' technique, and to the endocrine system in particular, is that each chakra can be said to have a physical counterpart with each gland. This reinforces the belief that the body is the emotions. Each gland is not only physical but also emotional. Modern Western scientific research has begun to find its own explanations for this phenomenon and Candace Pert, in her book 'Molecules of Emotion', says

> *'... the key concept is that the emotions exist in the body as informational chemicals, the neuropeptides and receptors, and they also exist in another realm, the one we experience as feeling, inspiration, love — beyond the physical. The emotions move back and forth, flowing freely between both places, and, in that sense, they connect the physical and non-physical. Perhaps this is the same thing that Eastern healers call the subtle energy, or prana — the circulation of emotional and spiritual information throughout the bodymind... My work has taught me that there is a physical reality to the emotions.'*

The endocrine 'links' can be held, with any imbalances being felt. It would be too prescriptive, too analytical, to focus on one specific link; the ideal approach is to work intuitively with the whole system, aiming for an even distribution of energy throughout. The body's own innate intelligence should be trusted and respected. Each energy centre does not exist in isolation; the entire system is interwoven and is constantly changing, reflecting its dynamics.

However, for reasons of clarity, in this chapter each gland is described in turn, although this is quite artificial as, with the body's remarkable ability, each one is constantly adjusting and responding to activity within its fellow glands. 'Linking' attempts, albeit it humbly, to support this connection. The non- physical presentation of this system can provide deeper understanding of an individual and a sense of direction emotionally within a treatment.

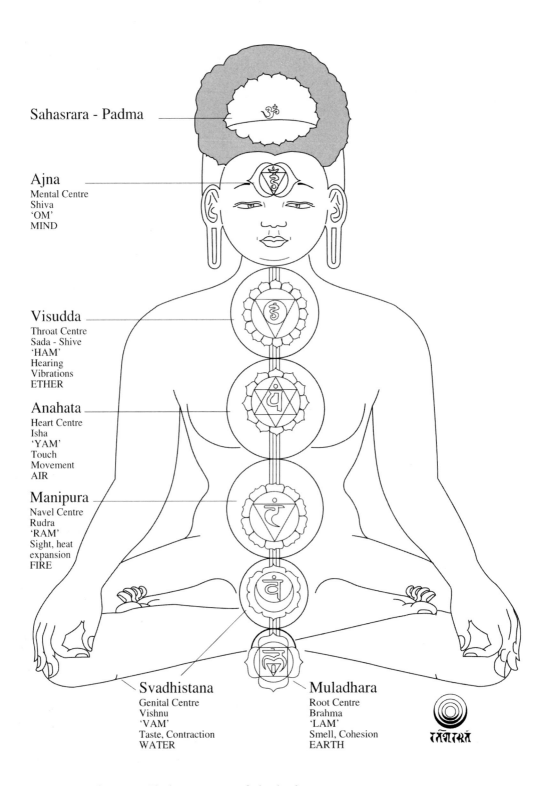

Sahasrara - Padma

Ajna
Mental Centre
Shiva
'OM'
MIND

Visudda
Throat Centre
Sada - Shive
'HAM'
Hearing
Vibrations
ETHER

Anahata
Heart Centre
Isha
'YAM'
Touch
Movement
AIR

Manipura
Navel Centre
Rudra
'RAM'
Sight, heat
expansion
FIRE

Svadhistana
Genital Centre
Vishnu
'VAM'
Taste, Contraction
WATER

Muladhara
Root Centre
Brahma
'LAM'
Smell, Cohesion
EARTH

Figure 3.1: The yoga Chakra centres of the body

Chakra chart

Chakra	Physical	Non-physical
Sahasrara (crown)	Pineal gland	Spiritual awareness
Ajna (third eye)	Pituitary gland	The connections between the emotions and the physical body
Vishuddi (throat)	Thyroid gland	Communication
Anahata (heart)	Thymus gland	Relationships
Manipura (solar plexus)	Pancreas	Confidence
Svadisthana (sacral)	Adrenal glands	Courage
Muladhara (base)	Gonads	Vitality

The links associated with the endocrine system are:

1. Thyroid gland to itself.
2. Parathyroid glands to themselves.
3. Pituitary gland to the adrenal gland.
4. Pineal gland to the base of the spine.
5. Pituitary gland to the adrenal and the thyroid glands (a 3-way link).

The linking technique reinforces the natural communication processes of this system. *Figure 3.2* shows the reflexes for the endocrine glands.

The thyroid link is located by holding the central point of the thyroid reflex on the plantar aspect with the thumb of one hand and the middle finger of the other hand holding a point immediately above on the dorsal aspect (see *Figure 3.3*). The dorsal point is held still while the remainder of the plantar thyroid reflex is worked across to the medial line and then back again.

The practitioner can have a strong pulsating or tingling sensation or, at the other end of the spectrum, a flat or dull response. The client can have a pulsing, rod-like feeling between the two points, and it can feel tender — in which case the pressure needs to be reduced. The light touch of a link is often more effective than deep pressure. This link can be equally effective for an under-active, or over-active thyroid state because it aims to restore balance. It can be helpful for clients with low energy levels or with any imbalances within the metabolic process. It assists the natural function of the thyroid — and parathyroid — gland, adjusting the levels of calcium in the blood and the bones. Therefore, in cases where the level of this vital mineral is compromised, eg. arthritis and osteoporosis, it can be given special attention.

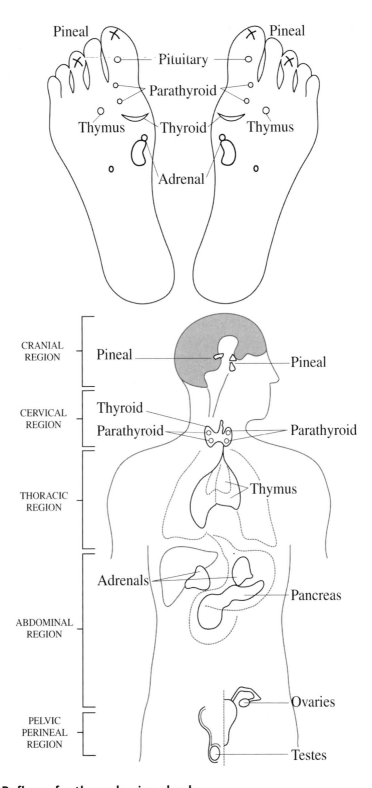

Figure 3.2: Reflexes for the endocrine glands

The parathyroid link is found by holding each plantar parathyroid reflex and linking it to itself with a dorsal point immediately above (see *Figure 3.4*). This can often feel hot for both the practitioner and the client, with the now familiar possibility of a rod-like connection through the foot. It has an invaluable application, along with the thyroid gland link, because of its ability to assist with the adjustment of calcium levels.

The pituitary gland is 'linked' to the adrenal by holding the pituitary with the thumb of one hand and the adrenal with the other thumb (see *Figure 3.5*). Often heat is felt on the adrenal reflex, and a feeling of connection between the two points. This appears to reinforce the natural communication between these two glands, and between the endocrine and nervous systems (because of the adrenal response to stressful situations). It can restore balance, having a beneficial effect on the nervous system and creating a feeling of deep relaxation. It has a specific application for menopausal women, assisting with hormonal balance and reducing the over activity of the menopausal adrenal gland, helping to reduce the severity and frequency of hot flushes. Adrenal energy can become depleted as a result of stress, hormonal imbalances or by the consumption of stimulants such as coffee or alcohol, and this energy can be revitalised by this link.

The pineal gland can be 'linked' to the base of the spine, simply by holding the pineal reflex with one thumb and the sacrum with the middle finger of the other hand (see *Figure 3.6*). The practitioner can feel this as a circuit of energy or as a sensation of lightening, of releasing. The client often says that this feels 'floaty' and relaxing. It is especially useful at the end of a treatment, as it both seals and closes down the session.

It is possible to apply three-way 'links', one of these being between the pituitary, adrenal and thyroid glands. It is located by holding the pituitary and adrenal glands as previously described and then taking the middle finger of one hand to hold the dorsal thyroid reflex (see *Figure 3.7*). This can feel very powerful, with both people feeling the strong triangle-like connection between the three points. There can be a feeling of heat, or sometimes a sensation of energy 'bouncing' from one point to another. It can establish a holding, secure feeling. It is often helpful when clients feel the need to release pent-up emotions. These anxieties may be recent or they may be long-standing, perhaps from childhood. Often the action of verbalising and releasing these concerns is therapeutic in itself. This release will only happen when the individual is ready but, if the practitioner can sense that this is the case, it can mimic the effect of giving someone a hug and allowing him/her to feel secure and safe within the emotional state. It is powerful, encompassing a major portion of a crucial system of the body.

Every system within the body is continually communicating and responding to each other, but the endocrine and nervous systems together have a unique role with the task of maintaining homeostasis, that state of balance that the body strives to be in.

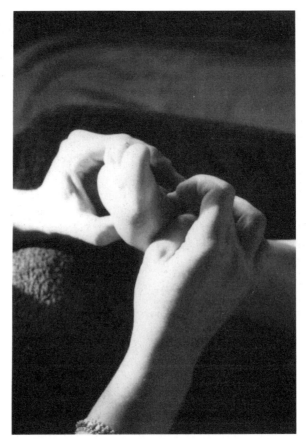

Figure 3.3

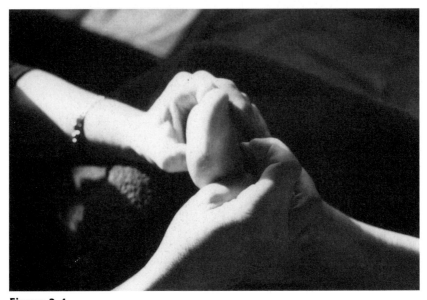

Figure 3.4

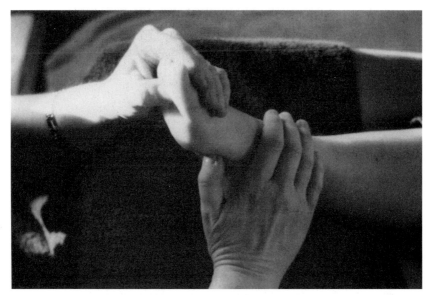

Figure 3.5

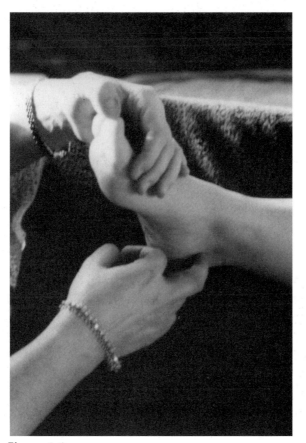

Figure 3.6

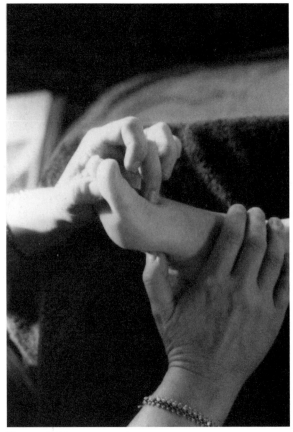

Figure 3.7

Taking into account the tremendous amount of both internal and external stresses in the modern world, this two-way relationship between hormone and tension levels is amazingly resilient, robust and effective. There is a constant feedback operating within the endocrine system, trying to maintain order. It is an all-powerful system having an effect on the entire body.

The endocrine system can be seen as the way in which we cope with our environment. It can reflect the level of harmony, within the self, and with the world. When there is an imbalance within this system it is often reported as a feeling of 'loss of control', or 'not coping'. It can feel like an all-encompassing process over which the individual has no control, and an imbalance can produce behaviour and feelings that are quite out of character. This can be, at best, confusing and, at worst, terrifying. Reflexology, at these times, can offer specific help with restoring balance and reducing stress levels. Perhaps, more importantly, the practitioner can also offer reassurance and support, and give realistic self-help advice so that individuals can begin to feel in control of themselves again.

Case studies

1. Client details — Hazel. Age 52. Married. One grown-up daughter. Runs local village shop.

Presenting symptom: Menopausal hot flushes. She feels that these dominate her life; she has several overnight, resulting in very disturbed sleep for herself and her husband. She also has frequent hot flushes during the day, sometimes so severe that she has to leave the room and go outdoors. These now restrict her social life. She is determined not to take HRT, wanting to manage the menopause naturally.

Treatment: On presentation all the endocrine and reproductive reflexes felt hot and tender. The neck area was tight with the neck to jaw link feeling very energetic to the practitioner, so this was held several times during the treatment. The pituitary to adrenal link was also worked, with heat felt on the adrenal. There was a steady improvement for the first four weekly sessions, with the heat on the adrenal reflex gradually reducing and, at the same time, Hazel felt that the night-time sweats were less severe. After the fourth treatment, the symptoms worsened for a short time but, after the sixth treatment, there continued to be a steady improvement. At this time, the hot flushes had reduced both in severity and frequency. The usual pattern is just one which she is aware of overnight but not enough to disturb her sleep, and perhaps two or three during the day but, as she says, 'they are manageable now'. She feels delighted and confident that she can allow the menopause to progress naturally and she has regular monthly treatments to sustain this improvement. She thoroughly enjoys the sessions and says that 'it does work but, even if it didn't, I would still come because it feels wonderful'.

Incidentially, she realised after several months that she had not needed to make the regular appointment with her osteopath because she had had no neck problems.

2. Client details — Joyce. Age 35. Married with three young children.

Presenting symptom: Premenstrual syndrome. This lasts for two weeks before each period when she feels irritable and depressed. This feels alien to her because she normally has a positive attitude to life. She feels tired 'all the time'.

Treatment: She was intrigued and fascinated by the full treatment she received which gave particular focus to the entire endocrine system. The thyroid reflex felt very dull and flat on the left foot. The pituitary to adrenal, thyroid and parathyroid links were all worked. The small intestines reflex was also tender and tight.

She received four weekly treatments, then the interval was extended to fortnightly for four more sessions, and then regular monthly sessions were established. After the sixth treatment, she felt an improvement in her overall energy levels and after three months she felt that there had been a gradual reduction in the severity of the PMS. This is now an occasional problem, not associated with every period and only lasting for three or four days. She values the consultation time as her only relaxation in a very busy schedule.

3. Client details — Josephine. Age 36. Single. Lives alone except for her small dog. No children. She is unemployed, having had to retire because of the state of her health.

Presenting symptoms: Myalgic encephalomyelitis (ME) for five years. She has disturbed sleep patterns, only being able to sleep for two or three hours at a time.

She tends to sleep both throughout the day and night and so has no social life. Her concentration levels are low and she feels that she has no energy at all. She experiences muscular pain and feels frustrated and uncoordinated because she wants to move but finds it hard, sometimes impossible, to do so.

Treatment: At the first treatment, the practitioner felt strong reactions with some of the links, namely the neck to jaw and lumbar 5 to hip ones. These were worked several times during the treatment although each time the client felt very little. She did feel that the pituitary reflex was tender so this was gently worked. The pressure throughout was very light and Josephine relaxed and fell asleep after thirty minutes. At the second treatment, one week later, Josephine reported feeling exceptionally tired after the initial treatment and had, in fact, slept for almost twenty four hours. She needed reassurance that, hopefully, this would not happen after every session. Attention was given to the pituitary/adrenal link with a view to boosting energy; this felt quite vibrant and the client felt a connection between the two reflexes which she described as a 'red, dotted line'. Again a strong reaction was felt by the practitioner on the neck/jaw and lumbar 5/hip links. Josephine relaxed and slept again. One week later, at the third treatment, she felt more positive in general and looked brighter. For two nights in the week she had slept for a longer period of time and was, therefore, awake for longer in the day-time. The pineal to base link was held with the aim to adjust melatonin levels. When the lumbar 5 to hip link was held, Josephine felt a connection between the two points and also felt a tingling sensation moving up her leg. She felt encouraged by this saying 'perhaps there is some life in my legs after all'.

The fourth treatment was two weeks later and Josephine looked more alert and was smiling. She was very pleased with herself having managed to walk her dog, instead of having to ask a neighbour and she was sleeping better with clearer distinctions between the day and night time. Again she felt some referred sensations with some of the links.

She continued with monthly treatments for three months and then settled to six-weekly sessions. The ME remains a major part of her life but she usually manages a daily walk and because of her adjusted sleep routine, she can organise a social life, albeit it quite limited. In appearance she continues to look brighter and smiles more. She still has periods of depression but feels that these are less severe. From time to time she talks about childhood problems, notably a difficult relationship with her father. She sees the reflexology consultations as a way of 'off loading' and helping her to cope. She has started to attend a Yoga class and is surprised by the benefits from this, both physical and emotional.

4. **Client details — Mabel. Age 67. Married. Busy. Loves organising.**

Presenting symptom: Arthritis in both knees.

Treatment: On presentation, the neck and shoulders were very tight and tense. The neck to jaw link was held and she commented that this felt uncomfortable. The thyroid and parathyroid links were also held with a view to increasing bone calcium levels. Mabel found it difficult to relax, she didn't close her eyes at all and talked throughout the session. She was interested in the effect of diet on her condition, this being a new concept for her, and she discussed with the practitioner how she could reduce acid-forming food realistically. At the second session her feet felt more relaxed, although the neck to jaw link was still powerful and tender. She was quiet for a short time. At the third treatment she talked about her granddaughter and then started to talk about herself as a child, about her brother and also about her very strict father who had often made her feel frightened and angry. As she talked, her feet, and the rest of her, began to relax. The pituitary to adrenal to thyroid link was being gently held and she seemed to soften and smiled more (instead of frowning).

At subsequent treatments, usually at monthly intervals, she relaxes after a short while and closes her eyes. The neck and shoulder reflexes became less tense each time. She has commented that it is 'wonderful just to be able to talk about myself'. She still has painful knees but she manages to enjoy her garden with some help and her overall appearance is brighter.

Reference

Pert CB (1998) *Molecules of Emotion*. Simon and Schuster, New York: 307

4
Framework

To attach meaning to the consultations, it is necessary to remember that two of the main functions of the skeleton are:

- protection
- movement.

If someone has a problem with the framework of their body they, understandably, feel vulnerable with a loss of protection and control. This is especially so if it is a spinal problem, with the person feeling that the very core of their being is damaged. Reduced movement produces feelings of frustration and depression and often the associated pain is debilitating in itself. These feelings can be addressed within the actual hands-on treatment; if a client is feeling depressed and low then a stimulating treatment to lift the spirits would be appropriate. The relationship between each person and the practitioner can also help emotionally. The aim is for the client to feel respected and cared for; in this supportive environment he/she can begin to feel in control of various aspects of his/her health. The manner and context of the dialogue need not be intense or daunting but, rather, relaxed and conversational in style. Some individuals may welcome an opportunity to discuss emotional problems, for others it may be more appropriate to discuss realistic ways to take charge of their own health in practical ways, eg. dietary changes or a gentle exercise programme. A positive outcome would be for the client to be involved in, and confident with, their own healthcare.

The 'links' influencing the skeletal system are:

- neck to jaw
- lumbar 5 to hip
- leg and arm work.

The whole length of the spine is worked (see *Figure 4.1*), using circular movements of the thumb or middle finger to locate the reflex for each vertebrae. Gentle yet effective pressure is used with particular attention being given to sensitive areas.

For any neck condition, pain and tension in the jaw or for tension headaches, the neck to jaw link can be used (see *Figure 4.2*). The reflex for cervical 5 is linked to the jaw reflex inside the big toe. This is particularly effective for people who have tension in their jaw, or who grind their teeth. It is an easy link to locate, with the practitioner often feeling a pulsating sensation on either or both of the points. Often heat is felt by the practitioner and/or the client. The client often reports feeling a connection running through, or around, the big toe. The importance of this link is that it is frequently painful to work directly on the neck reflex but, with a light touch, this technique is both effective and powerful.

A powerful link is lumbar 5 to hip reflex (see *Figure 4.3*). The 5th lumbar vertebrae reflex (on the medial aspect) is held and linked to the hip reflex (on the lateral aspect). This is particularly effective for any hip or knee conditions or for conditions affecting the sciatic nerve. It has a relaxing effect on the nervous system so it can be applied to any stress-related problems.

This can be amplified further by transferring it into a 3-way link by holding the mid-point of the sciatic loop on the plantar aspect (see *Figure 4.4*). This has a specific application for conditions affecting the sciatic nerve.

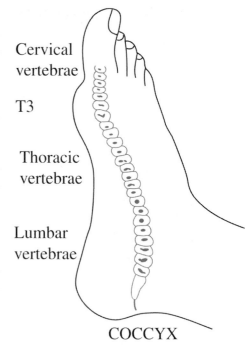

Cervical vertebrae

T3

Thoracic vertebrae

Lumbar vertebrae

COCCYX

Figure 4.1

This connection between the lumbar spine and the hip represents an area of the body that is full of activity, ie. the pelvis. The 'link' reflects the energetic sense of the client, sometimes with the practitioner feeling a strong, pulsating energy and sometimes a calm, light response. Neither is right or wrong but it matches the person at that time, with the aim being, as with all reflexology, to find a balance.

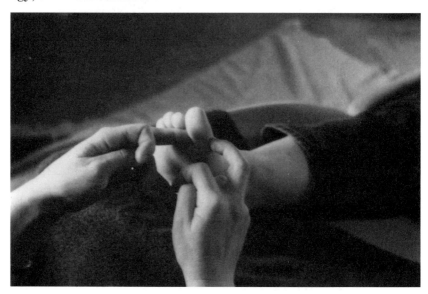

Figure 4.2

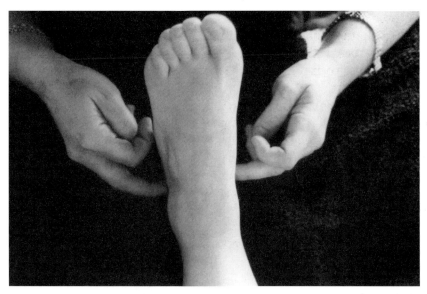

Figure 4.3

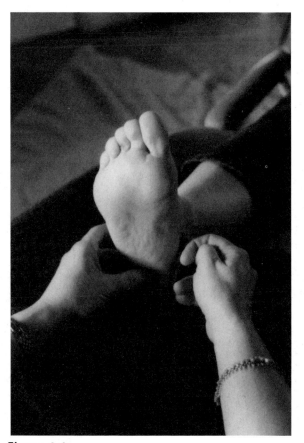

Figure 4.4

As with the neck/jaw link, the practitioner can feel heat and a sense of connection through the foot. The client can report feeling the same rod-like connection, also sometimes a tingling sensation moving up the leg, perhaps to the hip or into the spine. This tends to be directed to where it is most needed so, for instance, it may be described as a warmth moving around the knee or around the hip and then returning down again. The energy can regulate itself and fade away when appropriate — with both the client and the practitioner feeling this. Each person's reactions to the links are quite unique, with some people feeling referred reactions in the body and others feeling very little; neither is correct or incorrect but rather represents how that individual is functioning at that time. As clients relax into this procedure, the words that have been used to describe it include 'floating', 'lightening' and 'opening out' — these appear to be accurate ways of outlining a release of tension with our limited Western vocabulary. Often it can feel very comforting to have the foot held in this way.

Precision reflexology has an interesting procedure for working the reflexes for the legs and arms using the linking technique. The lumbar 5 reflex is held while the middle finger of the other hand traces the outline of the leg on the lateral aspect of the foot (see *Figure 4.5*).

The arm is worked by holding the point for thoracic 3 on the spinal reflex and linking across to the shoulder reflex on the lateral aspect of the foot (this can have positive results when treating shoulder problems such as 'frozen shoulder'). Then the arm reflex is tracked down to the wrist area. At this point the medial link is changed to cervical vertebrae 2 and the arm is tracked back up to the shoulder with the 'circuit' being completed by working across the foot to the jaw link (see *Figure 4.6*). The method for arm and leg work amplifies the effects of treatment.

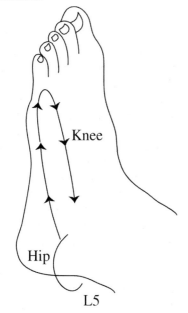

Figure 4.5

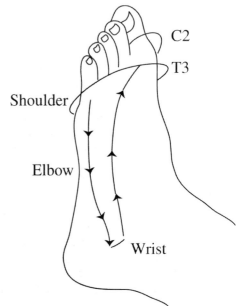

Figure 4.6

Within a treatment, the whole length of the spine is worked. Initially, the jaw link is held with the middle finger of one hand, as small circular pressure is applied along the cervical vertebrae with the middle finger of the other hand. Then the jaw link is released, and this finger is placed lightly on the top of the big toe, and remains there, while working along the length of the spine down to the coccyx. Then follows the leg and arm work as described above. Using linking to work the spine amplifies a treatment, increases sensitivity and often creates dramatic connections within the actual spine. Using small circular strokes, it is possible to detect precisely each individual vertebrae. Sensitive areas may reflect structural problems or neurological ones, often indicating an imbalance within an organ which has its nerve intervention at that point. At the tender spots, the reflex is held lightly in order to increase the effectiveness. This can be assisted by guiding the client through appropriate breathing techniques, to direct the breath to a particular area. Using this approach, the experienced practitioner can feel a variety of responses which match how that person is feeling. The information that can be picked up from this spinal work is significant, as it usually mirrors the nature of the client, with tender areas often reflecting emotion sensitivities.

Case study

Client details — James. Age 61. Retired clerical officer. Married.

Presenting symptom: Arthritis in his knees. When describing how he feels about this, he says that he feels 'cheated' because he was looking forward to enjoying an active retirement. He experiences pain and stiffness in the morning and he feels afraid to walk in case the pain levels increase.

Treatment: Obviously he received a full treatment at each session, with the focus on the solar plexus area for pain relief, on the adrenals in order to stimulate the body's natural anti-inflammatories and also (thinking about the fight/flight response) to address the feelings of fear. The primary 'links' would be the lumbar 5 to knee (as part of the procedure for working the leg reflex) and, also, the thyroid and parathyroid ones (see *Chapter 3*).
Initially James found it difficult to relax; he talked a lot during the first treatment and had his eyes open throughout. At this first consultation there was a realistic discussion about his health. He was not looking for, or expecting, a cure but he was reassured by a positive outlook of, hopefully, slowing down the progress of his condition. Dietary recommendations were also discussed, with the aim of reducing acid-forming foods, ie. concentrated proteins. He talked about realistic ways in which he could achieve this yet still have a diet that he would enjoy. To assist with the removal of toxins, and to improve his overall circulation, he was guided through a basic deep breathing routine. This approach was completely new to him but he felt much brighter and, in his words, 'at least there is something that I can do for myself'.
He was intrigued by the feel of the linking technique. The lumbar 5 to knee was an especially strong response and he described feeling a definite tingle in his knees. This in itself boosted his morale; he said that it reassured him that there was 'life in there still'.
After four fortnightly sessions, he feels that the pain is now reduced each morning. He feels

more confident and is taking gentle walks each day. During the treatments he now relaxes, closing his eyes. He is beginning to make plans for his retirement, talking with his wife about going on holiday and has started gardening again — with some help for the heavier jobs.

5
Movement

The muscles of the body provide strength and mobili⸱ ⸱roblems can
produce feelings of weakness, frustration, heaviness ⸱es, depression.
We can move from the day we are born and, when ⸱ ⸱s compromised,
naturally our spirits can be deeply affected. A⸱ ⸱ described, these
feelings can be addressed in the more non-specif⸱ ⸱f the consultation.

    For some conditions it can be very th⸱ ⸱n the acute stage, to
realise the benefit of rest with a gradual in⸱ ⸱of gentle exercise. This
process alone often allows the person conce⸱ ⸱rn to care for him/herself
with awareness.

    Just as the feet represent the ⸱ ⸱the whole body, the entire
muscular system has reflex points on ⸱ ⸱see *Figure 5.1*). In a standard
treatment the whole of the foot is wor⸱ ⸱scribed in *Chapter 13*) and all the
muscles are given attention. The ⸱ ⸱r the muscles of the spine can be
specifically worked by applying ⸱ ⸱1umb pressure to either side of the
spinal reflex for its full length.

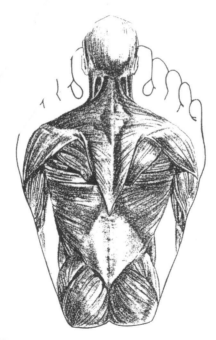

Figure 5.1

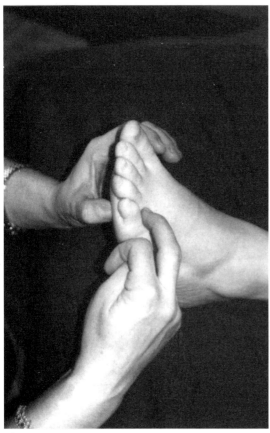

Figure 5.2

The specific link for this system is:

- shoulder link — plantar reflex through to dorsal (see *Figure 5.2*).

A reflex point at the base of the 4th toe on the plantar aspect is held using one thumb, with the middle finger of the other hand holding a point immediately above on the dorsal aspect. This is effective for muscular problems of the shoulder area. Often both the practitioner and the client feel heat with this link and either, or both, may be aware of a rod-like connection through the foot. The client may need reassurance with this feeling and deep breathing exercises practised at the same time can be beneficial.

Emphasising the importance of every aspect of the spine, the muscles here are involved with the overall health of the person. When treating a client who presents with a shoulder or arm condition, the practitioner can often feel tension and restriction in the reflex for the thoracic muscles. Likewise, with a client who has a pelvic or leg problem, a similar response can be felt in the lumbar reflexes. This is one of the strengths of reflexology, in that it can help to find the root cause of a problem. Often, when working the reflexes for the spinal muscles, a client's breathing will deepen and they become more relaxed, thus assisting with the overall situation.

Case study

Client details — Norma. Age 47. Married with two children (one married daughter and one son at university). She cares for her elderly mother who is becoming increasingly dependent. She is a teacher, which she used to enjoy, but she is now dissatisfied with this and says 'this is not the job that I trained to do'.

Presenting symptoms: Pain in her left shoulder. Headaches, which she herself feels are a result of the shoulder tension.

Treatment: On presentation, both right and left shoulder reflexes were tight and tender with this being more pronounced on the left side. She obviously received a full treatment with particular areas of tension being the solar plexus, the neck and the small intestine. The muscular shoulder 'link' was held through the foot. Gentle pressure was applied and this link was repeated several times during the treatment. The neck to jaw link (see *Chapter 4*) was also used; this being a very light touch as this area was tender. All the reflexes around the head area were very erratic and a focus within the session was to calm these down.

She valued this time for herself and felt that she had been given 'permission to be still' for one hour — which she described as 'bliss'.

After the first treatment the shoulder pain worsened for two days and then eased. This was followed by three further consultations, at weekly intervals, after which time the shoulder pain remained consistently reduced and the headaches were less frequent and less severe. She continues to attend at monthly intervals and the relationship between her and the practitioner has developed into one of mutual trust and respect. Her observations have progressed from saying 'it is so wonderful to have nothing to do for one hour' to a realisation of the benefits of relaxation spilling over into her own time. After three months, she made a conscious decision to care for herself, justifying this by saying it is the least she can do because she feels so cared for during the treatments. Consultation dialogue had centred around appropriate nutrition and the importance of not eating when stressed or hurried, so she set aside time to eat lunch. This involved the co-operation of her colleagues who, incidentally, have started to follow her example. She now attends a weekly keep-fit class, both for the exercise and to give her some time for herself.

She has arranged part-time care for her mother and has come to terms with this, having described to the reflexologist her understandable, but groundless, feelings of guilt and inadequacy. She now accepts that she had previously felt overwhelmed with responsibility, but this is now much reduced as she has begun to share these feelings with her husband. So, literally, she has lessened some of the burden from her shoulders.

6

Communication

The nervous system is the body's communication network, sending messages around to its various parts. Not surprisingly, when people under stress describe themselves as 'living on their nerves', or feeling 'nervy', they feel out of control and not connected within themselves or with their environment. The treatment provides an opportunity to break the stress pattern, to go into a state of relaxation. Given time, hopefully, the benefits can extend outside the treatment room and the individual can achieve a sense of control in daily life.

A full reflexology treatment has a beneficial effect on the entire nervous system, promoting deep relaxation: bringing obvious benefits to clients who are experiencing any stress-related problems.

The specific link for this system is:

- forebrain to sacrum.

One thumb holds the forebrain area on the big toe, while the middle finger of the other hand holds the sacrum (see *Figure 6.1*). In effect, the conscious thinking part of the brain is connected to the base of the spine. It is ideal for people who find it difficult to unwind and to 'switch off' their thoughts. It aims to take the person into a parasympathetic nervous state, facilitating relaxation, creating an optimum situation for the body to heal itself and to strive for homeostasis. Often, for clients who chatter nervously, this link has been known to silence them in mid-sentence. Practitioners can sometimes feel an imbalance between these two points and be aware of a sense of release as the forebrain area calms down. Clients describe this 'link' as feeling 'floaty, 'calming' and a 'draining away' of tension.

Every treatment begins by holding the solar plexus reflex and, in this way, gaining an insight into the nervous state of the person. At this point, it is possible to detect levels of stress, pain and anxiety. For instance, it can feel energetic or dull, delicate or robust, vibrant or calm — all reflecting that person in a neurological manner.

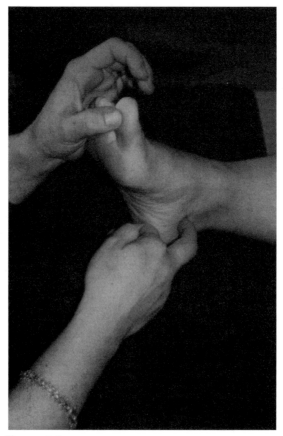

Figure 6.1

Case study

Client details — Phyllis. Age 42. Married with two sons aged eleven and thirteen. Her husband works away from home during the week. She is a personel officer who carries a high level of both responsibility and stress.

Presenting symptoms: Headaches. She feels that these are mainly stress-related. Pre-menstrual syndrome, the worst aspect of this being intense irritability.
Weight gain. She believes this to be hormonal and she has an uncontrollable sugar craving associated with the PMS. She is very organised and controlled with all other areas of her life and she feels 'ashamed' about this.
She is a bright, extrovert personality, is aware of the stress factors in her life and of how these may be affecting her present state of health.

Treatment: On presentation, the thyroid and neck reflexes were tender, reflecting her tension and the forebrain reflex area felt very erratic and tingly to the practitioner. Over a period of time it has become more responsive until now, although at the beginning of every session it still feels powerful (as it needs to be for Phyllis' life-style) it becomes calmer as the link with the sacrum is held.
The first three treatments were at fortnightly intervals and, then there were regular

monthly sessions. She enjoyed the treatments immediately but did not relax until the third session. After the first two treatments the headaches worsened and then, after the third, they were noticeably reduced, both in severity and frequency. The irritability associated with the PMS has steadily reduced and she now feels that it is manageable.

Within the consultation, she discussed her eating patterns. In order to maintain a steady blood-sugar level, she has organised herself to take time to eat breakfast and a piece of fruit mid-morning (instead of the previous chocolate bar). She now leaves her desk so that she eats in a relaxed manner at lunch time. This has eliminated the need for a 'quick hit' of sugar in the afternoon, and then she has a small evening meal. In addition, also considering the blood-sugar levels, she has gradually reduced her coffee intake. The sugar cravings are far less frequent now. Previously, if she succumbed to the cravings, she felt guilty and, if she resisted them, then she had a sense of denial. Now, if she does eat chocolate, she can enjoy it, knowing that it is an occasional treat. As a result, her self-esteem is restored.

She continues with monthly treatments, feeling the benefit of the 'time-out' in a very busy life. She reports handling stressful situations in a calmer manner.

7
Fuel

The functions of the digestive system are ingestion, digestion, absorption, assimiliation and elimination of food. It is affected by stress in a very instinctive, primitive way. The intestines have a strong relationship with the nervous system and with the emotions — we have all experienced the phenomenon of a 'gut feeling' so it could be said that the intestines are themselves emotional when feelings of tension or excitement are felt in this area. Unfortunately, modern Westerners generally abuse this system with an over-refined, inadequate diet, often ignoring its 'messages' concerning the effect of stress in their lives. The body is not designed to digest food when in a 'fight/flight' situation, as other functions of the body are more necessary. The Eastern approach, which says that if you eat when angry, stressed or hurried then the food is a poison, bears this out.

Eating fresh, whole food is one way of taking charge of one's own health. Also, by responding to the information from the digestive process, for example eating only when hungry and resting the system when necessary, demonstrates an awareness of 'listening' to the body's messages and of caring for oneself accordingly.

Currently there is much confusion and emotion surrounding food issues. Clients often feel overwhelmed with information and they need reassurance and guidance just to remind them that, primarily, eating ought to be an enjoyable and social event — which can also be nutritious.

The reflexes for the digestive system are shown in *Figure 7.1*. The specific link is:

- gall bladder to itself.

The gall bladder reflex is held with the thumb of one hand, with the middle finger of the other hand holding a point immediately above on the dorsal aspect of the foot (see *Figure 7.2*).

This can improve the function of the gall bladder, aiding the digestion of fat. It is especially helpful in reducing tension within the entire digestive process.

The stomach reflex is given attention with a circular thumb stroke to cover the whole area. Generally speaking, this organ is quite robust and therefore a firm pressure can be applied — unless the recipient has a stomach disorder, or if it feels tender to touch, when appropriate sensitivity should be used.

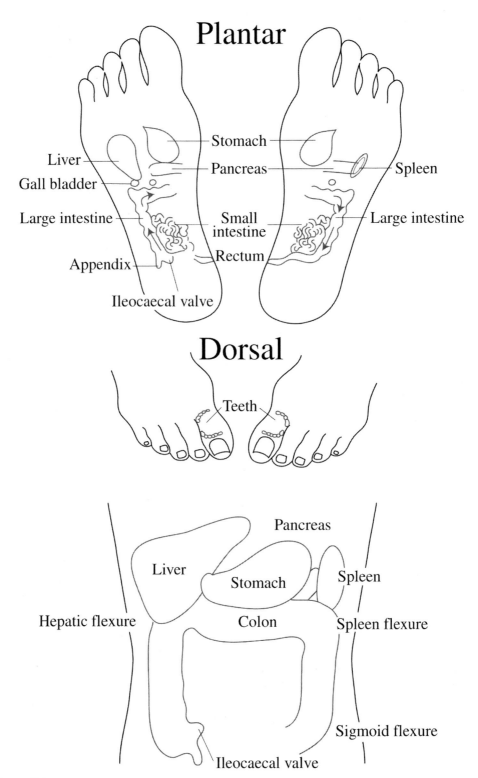

Plantar

Stomach
Liver
Pancreas
Spleen
Gall bladder
Large intestine
Small intestine
Large intestine
Rectum
Appendix
Ileocaecal valve

Dorsal

Teeth

Pancreas
Liver
Stomach
Spleen
Hepatic flexure
Colon
Spleen flexure
Sigmoid flexure
Ileocaecal valve

Figure 7.1

The same approach applies to the liver reflex, firm thumb pressure being used to cover the reflex area unless otherwise indicated. For variety, a different stroke can be used to cover the small intestine reflex. One that is pleasant to give and to receive is a 'fanning' stroke, with both thumbs working horizontally across the foot from side to side, one above the other (see *Figure 7.3*). Also, in order to 'scan' the relatively large area of the intestines, a 'walking' stroke can be used. This involves moving diagonally over the area with the thumb, the pressure being constant with the joint remaining soft as the thumb glides along (see *Figure 7.4*). This can often indicate where more attention is needed and this can then be given with the more specific circular thumb pressure. To cover the large intestine reflex this, now familiar, circular thumb stroke is used to move along its length.

As you would expect, the nature of the intestinal reflexes often reflects the emotional state of the client, for instance, they can feel tense and congested or flexible and relaxed.

Case study

Client details — Mavis. Age 32. She is a single parent with two children aged four and two. She is a full-time mother.

Presenting symptom: Irritable bowel syndrome. She experiences abdominal pain and bloating. She has a very restricted diet and feels miserable about this. She is slightly overweight.

Treatment: Mavis' initial reaction was one of delight because of having time to herself, to be 'pampered' as she said. She received a full treatment, with gentle attention to the small and large intestine both of which felt very tight and tender. The gall bladder link was held lightly, with the practitioner feeling intense heat. The client relaxed instantly and fell asleep for a short time.

After three treatments, at monthly intervals, she reported that the pain and bloating were both reduced; each time the intestines felt looser and the heat on the gall bladder reduced. At the fourth session, she was quite tearful and talked about her feelings of loss and loneliness since her divorce, which she had been unable to express before.

In order to relax and to improve the circulation to the intestines, the reflexologist guided Mavis through deep breathing exercises which she practices daily at home. Also, to improve abdominal tone and to reduce weight, she has included some exercises into this daily routine that fit in with her home life, either being a walk with the children or by using a video tape.

She continues with regular monthly treatments. The feet usually show neck and shoulder tension as well as the tight abdominal area, but all of these relax during the session. She has also been able to extend her diet and has completely pain-free spells.

There are occasional lapses which coincide with stressful times but these respond positively to the treatment.

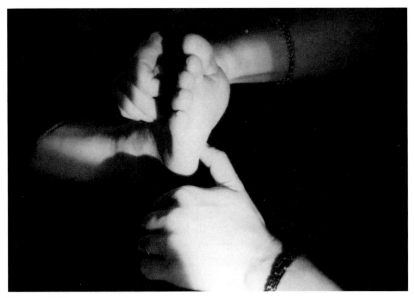

Figure 7.2

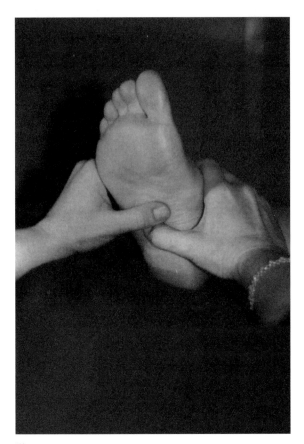

Figure 7.3

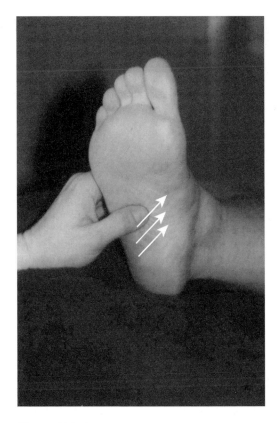

Figure 7.4

8

Vital energy

For people with severe respiratory conditions it is important to consider the emotional effects of the problem. We can survive for a considerable time without food and for several days without water, but only for a few minutes without breathing. If someone has breathing difficulties they feel, understandably, fearful and tense. Deep breathing exercises can address the problem both physically and emotionally. The exercises themselves, via the action of the diaphragm, massage the lungs and improve the circulation. There is a positive effect on the nervous system, with a reversal of the stress response, and the body being taken from the sympathetic into the parasympathetic state. Psychologically, the benefits can be huge with the client being aware of a real sense of self-control, with no external intervention.

It can also be helpful to pay attention to the client's posture and to gently guide them, with hands-on support, to sit tall with relaxed, wide shoulders. Sometimes people with restricted breathing unconsciously adopt a self-protective stance of rounded shoulders, without being aware that it has happened. This reduces the lung capacity still further but, by simply correcting posture, breathing can be improved. Also, emotionally, spirits can be raised by sitting tall and confidently looking forward.

The reflex areas for the respiratory system are shown in *Figure 8.1*. The associated link is :

- any tender lung area linked across to the spine.

For this link, any tender point which is found on the lung reflex area, either plantar or dorsal, is held with the thumb of one hand and then the other thumb is taken directly across to the spinal reflex on the medial line (see *Figure 8.2*).

Often heat is felt by the client, either on the reflex or in the actual lungs. Taking the tenderness across to the nerve intervention on the spine seems to relax the affected area, improving circulation and releasing tension.

The lungs in general are worked by applying pressure down the centre of the lung reflex area (both dorsal and plantar) and then spreading out the thumbs to each side of the foot. This creates a feeling of expansion and often encourages the client to breathe deeper.

The respiratory system is one of the body's eliminatory mechanisms. If there are respiratory problems there can also be tenderness in the digestive reflex areas, this being another way in which the body eliminates. Reflexology working on either of these two systems can indirectly benefit the other.

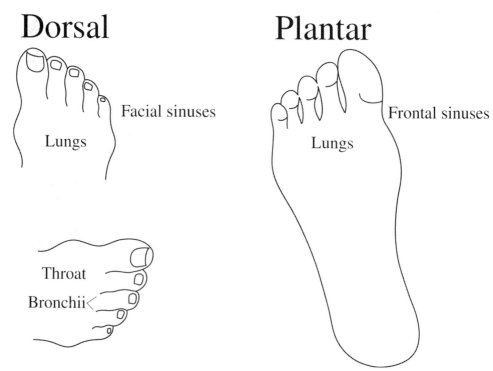

Dorsal

Facial sinuses

Lungs

Throat

Bronchii

Plantar

Frontal sinuses

Lungs

Figure 8.1

As a client relaxes during a treatment, breathing patterns noticeably change, becoming deeper and calmer. This provides an internal massage to the entire viscera. Depending on the nature of the client, and to restore a sense of balance, it may be more appropriate to advise calming breathing techniques on the one hand or, alternatively, energising ones on the other.

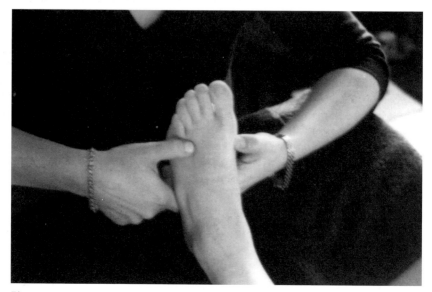

Figure 8.2

Case studies

1. Client details — Christine. Age 49. Head teacher of a large school. Obviously this is a responsible position with high stress levels. She enjoys her job but often feels stressed and, because she has to work most evenings and some weekends, she usually feels very tired.

Presenting symptom: Chronic painful sinusitis.

Treatment: On presentation the whole of the sinus reflexes were very tender. The pituitary and parathyroid areas were also painful. The ileo-caecal valve reflex was tender and felt hot to touch.

After four weekly treatments, the client reported having a very runny nose for two days and then being aware of noticeably reduced congestion, in her words 'the best for a long time'. After this the practitioner was able to apply stronger pressure as the sinus reflexes became less tender. At this time the client was also advised to reduce her intake of dairy food because of their mucous-forming properties and after the sixth treatment there were just isolated tender sinus points.

The treatments were reduced to monthly sessions and, after a further three sessions, the reflexes were completely free, as were the actual sinuses. It was discussed at this time, because the presenting symptom had now been addressed, that she may want to discontinue treatment, just returning as and when necessary. However, Christine felt that because the treatment had helped in other ways, namely reducing her stress levels and improving her overall immunity, she should continue on a monthly basis. She maintains that she 'needs to be given permission to switch off'.

Incidentally, she was concerned about her weight gain and, after several months into the course of treatment, she said 'after all this attention, the least I can do is to look after myself' so she joined a local exercise class, reduced her food intake and took the time to stop and eat lunch. She now has her weight under control.

2. Client details — James. Age 44. Married with two teenage children. Computer technician.

Presenting symptom: Bronchitis. He had never experienced this before. He looked pale, tired and drawn.

Treatment: Several points over the lung area felt tender and each of these was linked across to the spine. Each time both points felt hot for the practitioner. Also, James was guided through simple deep breathing exercises. His shoulder areas were tight and tender and particular attention was given to the lymphatic system with a view to assisting the body's protective mechanism. James relaxed during the treatment and his breathing eased.

He received four weekly treatments during the acute stage of his condition as he found this whole illness experience painful and frightening and wanted to make sure it didn't happen again. So, as a preventative measure, and because he enjoys them, he continues to practice deep breathing exercises at home, guided by a relaxation tape.

9

Nourishment

The function of this system is to transport nourishment around to every part of the body. When a person feels cold and tired, either physically or emotionally, it can be a sign that the circulation is sluggish. Every part of the body needs an effective blood supply for correct functioning and, as circulation benefits enormously by movement, so clients can help themselves with the introduction of appropriate exercise into their lifestyle.

Reflexology directly connects with the body's circulation, touching the extremities of this all-important system on the hands and the feet. In traditional Chinese medicine the quality of the blood and circulation is a primary diagnostic sign of health and illness. The Nei Ching states that the pulse can be,

> '... sharp as a hook, fine as a hair, taut as a musical string, dead as a rock, smooth as a flowing stream or as continuous as a string of pearls.'

(Majno, 1975)

It is interesting to note that these words quite accurately describe the sensitive responses often felt during a reflexology treatment. Much more accurately, in fact, than Western words that often seem to be too analytical and measured. During a standard full reflexology treatment the whole of the body's circulation is stimulated and improved. The specific link for the circulatory system is:

- adrenal reflex linked to the groin reflex.

This link is located by holding the adrenal reflex with the thumb of one hand and, with the middle finger of each hand, connecting to the groin reflexes (see *Figure 9.1*).

This three-way link can feel powerful with a sense of connection between the three points and often heat is felt on the adrenal area. It can be especially beneficial for clients with sluggish circulation, having a stimulating effect. It also appears to be beneficial as an added 'boost' for the adrenal gland in helping to restore salt and water balance in the body in cases of fluid retention.

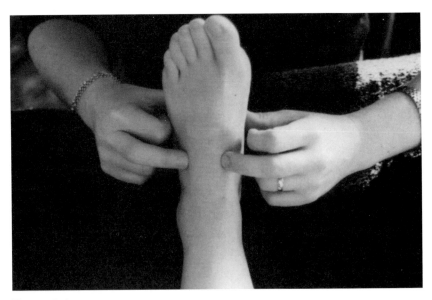

Figure 9.1

Case studies

1. Client details — Harry. Age 67. Widower. Retired.

Presenting symptom: Diabetic. He manages this condition well but is concerned about poor circulation in his feet.

Treatment: On presentation his feet are pale and extremely cold to touch. They became pinker and warmer in response to foot massage. During the treatment the adrenal to groin link was held several times on each foot. The adrenal point felt very tender — in fact, he instinctively pulled his foot away — so a light touch was used.
He received regular monthly treatments and, after the third one, he reported that his feet felt warmer and that they stayed warmer for longer periods of time. This has remained so, with monthly treatments in the winter and bi-monthly ones in the summer. His toes usually feel numb initially but warm up during the session. His poor circulation can still be a problem in the winter, but there has been no worsening of the situation despite his diabetes. During the consultation he often talks fondly about his late wife. He is obviously lonely and misses her terribly; he doesn't become upset but seems to enjoy the opportunity to reminisce.

2. Client details — Audrey. Age 52. After a long history of spinal problems, she had surgery several years ago which resulted in fusion of the lumbar vertebrae. She is realistic about her limitations and manages to have a full and active life. Married with three grown-up children.

Presenting symptom: Poor circulation and night-time cramps.

Treatment: She receives regular monthly treatments. After the second session she reported that the cramps were less frequent. She is very responsive throughout the treatment. Whenever the pituitary reflex is worked she feels a slight pulsing sensation in her temples; when the lumbar 5 to hip link is held she feels a 'floating and heavy sensation, as though waves are passing over' her. At the same time, the practitioner feels a charge of energy through her own arms. The adrenal to groin link often produces slight palpitations in Audrey's chest which feel strange but not unpleasant; she breathes deeply and the feeling subsides.

After the fourth treatment, Audrey said that her feet and legs were warmer and the cramp was much improved, with some nights being totally free. Two months later she was thrilled, saying that her feet were now warmer than her husband's, and her overall circulation has improved. She has regular treatments at six-weekly intervals and the improvement has been sustained.

Recently, as she greeted the practitioner, she announced proudly 'I feel so good about myself'.

Reference

Majno G (1975) *The Healing Hand: Man and Wound in the Ancient World*. Cambridge MA, Harvard University Press: 245

10
Reproduction

This sensitive system, perhaps more than any other, reflects inevitable life changes whether these be physical, emotional, social or lifestyle. This area of the body may alter the way that it has previously functioned, as though it mirrors the associated emotions presented by the new, challenging situation. The reflexes for the reproductive system are shown in *Figure 10.1*.

The links associated with this system are:

- ovary linked to uterus
- ovary to uterus to pituitary gland — a three-way link.

To locate the ovary to uterus link, hold the uterus reflex on the medial aspect of the foot with the middle finger of one hand and the ovary reflex on the lateral aspect with the middle finger of the other hand (see *Figure 10.2*). The ovary reflex can be held still while the uterus is worked with circular thumb pressure.

In order to reinforce the natural process within the endocrine system, this two-way link can be connected to the pituitary gland. To do this, the middle finger stays on the ovary but now the thumb of the same hand holds the uterus so that the other thumb can locate the pituitary reflex as in *Figure 10.3*.

These links can obviously be used for any problems with menstruation. The three-way link is particularly effective for any conditions involving irregularity in the menstrual cycle, for helping to restore a sense of balance and, also, for conditions associated with stress. Taking into account contraindications (see *Chapter 13*), these links should not be used during pregnancy.

Both these links often feel soft and delicate; a light touch being the most appropriate. Vibrations can be felt through the foot, or, with the three-way link, contained within a triangle of energy around the pelvic reflexes. Interestingly, especially for this particular system, clients report a feeling of being held or cradled. This also supports the emotional state that accompanies any disorders of this system.

The manner in which a person is not well, ie. the presenting symptom, often reflects how they are feeling emotionally and conditions affecting the reproductive system are no exception to this. It is no coincidence that the menopause, commonly referred to as 'the change', when a woman's reproductive cycle begins to alter, happens at a time of major lifestyle developments such as children leaving home, parents becoming dependant and possible career moves. These situations are not necessarily better or worse but certainly they are different and challenging and, inevitably, they call for emotional changes. Often an awareness of this connection creates a positive situation which supports a natural progression. There is less emphasis on an individual symptom and more on self-help and support mechanisms.

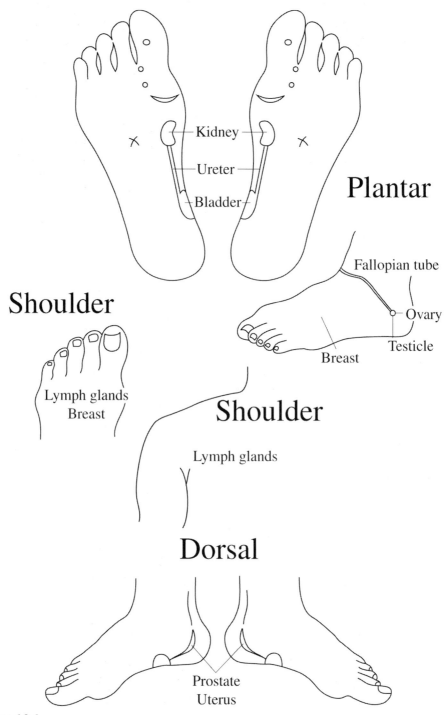

Figure 10.1

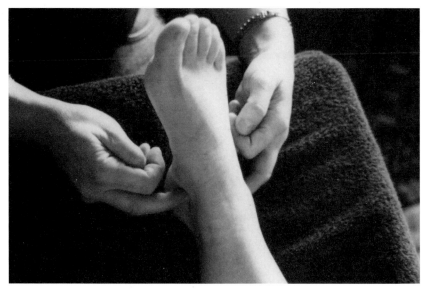

Figure 10.2

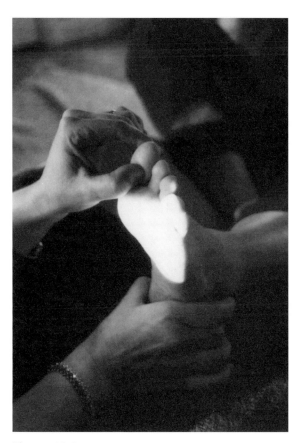

Figure 10.3

Case study

Client details — Alison. Age 28. Married. No children but she and her husband are wanting to start a family. Nurse.

Presenting symptoms: Irritable bowel syndrome. She experiences spells of abdominal bloating and diarrhoea. Endometriosis. This has only been diagnosed recently; over the last six months she has had heavy and painful periods. She often feels tired.

Treatment: On presentation there was a high degree of tension in the neck reflex, a very strong reaction on the pituitary reflex and the right ovary was very sensitive. The small and large intestines felt tight on both feet. Alison received a full treatment, the aim being to reduce overall stress levels, and special attention was given to the endocrine system in an attempt to restore balance. She fell asleep quickly but this appeared to be tiredness rather than relaxation.

At the first two sessions, the ovary to uterus link was held lightly, but this made the practitioner's fingers ache and the client felt heat on the ovary reflex. Thereafter, this was converted into the three-way link by also holding the pituitary reflex. The sensation of heat on the ovary was reduced and Alison described 'a pulse feeling moving between the three points'.

After four fortnightly appointments, the neck tension was considerably reduced, the overall response was calmer and her periods have, in her words, 'settled down'. The intestinal reflexes feel softer and she appears to be free of the IBS symptoms. After a further three monthly treatments, her menstrual cycle has reverted back to how it was before the endometriosis diagnosis. She is noticeably calmer, brighter and more relaxed generally. Since starting the course of treatment she has begun to attend a weekly Yoga class.

NB: The client at this time became pregnant. She continued with the Yoga classes but not with reflexology due to work commitments. She and her husband now have a beautiful baby daughter.

11
Protection

This system has a cleansing and protecting effect on the body. When it is struggling, it is a true case of lack of harmony with the environment, either internally within the body or externally with the world. Clients report feeling vulnerable, using phrases like 'if there is an infection around then I'll get it'. Reassurance and a positive attitude within the dialogue of the consultation are often valuable in themselves.

Reflexology, with its direct contact with lymphatic structures of the body, can have a powerful effect on this system. Care should be taken not to detoxify a highly toxic person too quickly, but rather to do this gradually in an acceptable way that can be maintained.

Practical, realistic changes to diet and exercise can improve lymphatic function and increase the body's protection. Also, this self-help approach can promote feelings of being empowered and, in this way, lift a person's spirits. Dietary recommendations involve receiving energy and protection from fresh, whole, untreated foods (see *Chapter 14*).

The lymphatic fluid requires movement in order to be able to travel through the body. Therefore exercise, in ways that are realistic and enjoyable for each individual, is vital.

The movement of lymphatic fluid that can result from a reflexology treatment is reflected in the way that recipients often describe themselves as feeling 'lighter' after such treatment.

The specific reflexes for the lymphatic system are shown in *Figure 11.1*. However, during a full treatment, the function of the lymph system is improved by the direct action of the foot massage.

The specific link for this system is:

- the thymus gland is linked to itself.

This is achieved by holding the thymus reflex (on the plantar aspect of each foot) with one thumb and then, with the middle finger of the other hand, holding a point immediately above on the dorsal aspect (see *Figure 11.2*). Often heat is felt, with a sense of connection through the foot. Alternatively, if a person's immune system is compromised, then it can feel flat and lifeless. In this way it can be used to boost immunity if appropriate to do so. At times of stress it can be helpful to give the thymus added attention; this gland has a vital role in that it matures 'T' cells (these form part of the body's immune processes) and this function is impaired when the body is under stress.

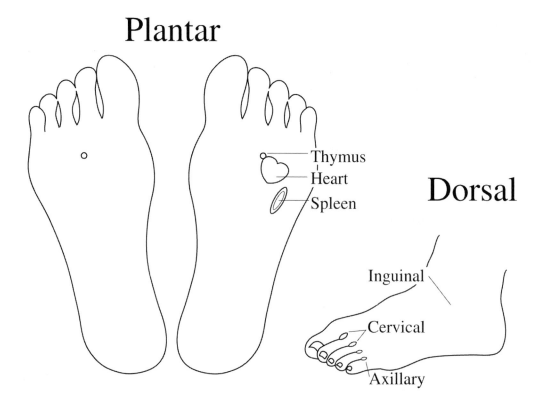

Figure 11.1

When the lymph system is sluggish, resulting in fluid retention, it can be beneficial to give attention to the urinary system during the treatment . This can involve using the pituitary to adrenal link referred to in *Chapter 7*. As an addition to this link, the pituitary remains held while working down from the adrenal gland reflex to the urether onto the bladder, then back to the adrenal gland. This appears to assist the body in restoring its salt/water balance.

Within a treatment, the most effective way of improving lymphatic function is with effleurage, massage strokes, working towards the heart. The lymphatic system can become sluggish for a variety of reasons, including illness, injury, trauma, poor nutrition, the effect of pollution, lack of exercise, medication, infection or stress. It has been proven that stress directly affects the body's level of immunity. In the 1980s Drs Jan and Ron Glaser, in America, conducted studies to find out if stress could have any effect on the cells of the immune system. They set up a controlled experiment using a group of medical students facing the stress of exams. They took blood samples from the students and measured the activity of white blood cells; key cells of the body's defence against disease. They found out that, immediately after the exams, the students had less active white blood cells. In 1988 they studied the effect of long-term low level stress on the immune and endocrine function. They studied married couples who described their marriages as

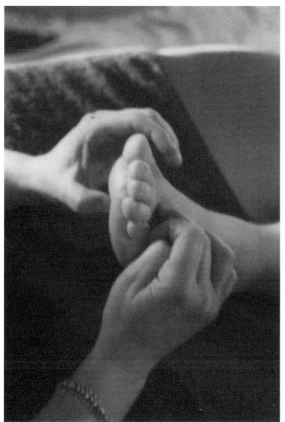

Figure 11.2

'poor'. The results showed that the wives' immune systems were weakened more significantly and for longer than their husbands'; the women found arguing more stressful than the men. This marital conflict study showed that chronic unrelenting stress did have a continuous dampening effect on the cells of the immune system. The Glasers also conducted a detailed study on carers with relatives who have Alzheimer's disease to monitor the effect on health of continuous high stress. The findings showed that in these people the immune response was lowered; the wounds of over-stressed carers took 24% longer to heal than did those of unstressed people. As a result of its ability to promote relaxation, it can be seen that reflexology will have a positive effect on the immune system.

Case study

Client details — Jean. Age 39. Married with two small sons.

Presenting symptoms: Fluid retention. Puffy hands and feet pre-menstrually. This can be so severe at times that she says her fingers look like 'sausages', she cannot bend them and, sometimes, cannot even pick up a cup.
Underactive thyroid gland. Overweight. She feels heavy and 'weighty'.

Treatment: She received a full treatment with particular attention to lymphatic drainage and to the thyroid gland. All the lymph reflexes were very tender to touch so light effleurage strokes were applied; the reflexes for the entire endocrine system were also very painful to touch. The thyroid link to itself was used; this felt very tingly to the practitioner and to Jean it felt warm and ached. The thymus link felt flat and lifeless. Throughout the treatment effleurage strokes to help drain the lymphatic fluid were repeated.
At the first session Jean enjoyed the time to focus on herself and to talk about her concerns regarding her weight. She knows that she lacks the time and the motivation to diet and exercise. Immediately after the treatment, and all subsequent ones, she needed to rush to the toilet. After the initial three weekly sessions, she reported frequent urination for the following twenty-four hours and extreme tiredness. During this time she had a period and

was amazed that she had no fluid retention. She has not lost any weight at all but feels 'lighter'.

The treatments were reduced to fortnightly for a further two months. The tiredness after the sessions ceased and the fluid retention became minimal. The thymus link now felt energetic. This remains the case, except when Jean is tired or stressed and then the link is held for a longer time until the energy is felt. She now felt ready to address the weight problem, she discussed a diet to fit in with her lifestyle and activity levels and also joined a local gym.

The treatments are now at monthly intervals, she feels supported by the consultations and reports back with progress of her weight loss. Nine months after the first session, she said 'I can now look at myself in the mirror without cringing'. She continues with regular treatments, with occasional problems with fluid retention but these are easily corrected. She continues to enjoy the 'time-out'.

12
Sensations

Our senses are the way in which we absorb information from our environment for interpretation. Understandably, if this is restricted in any way, then we feel isolated, vulnerable, depressed and often frightened. The reflexology consultation provides an ideal forum in which to offer support and reassurance. The reflexes for these areas are delicate and sensitive, as are the organs themselves, therefore the touch required needs to be equally light, sensitive and reassuring. There are no specific reflexes for the vital sense of touch but, obviously, this receives direct benefits during a treatment and, indirectly, by the positive effect on the entire nervous system.

The therapeutic benefits of touch, physiological and emotional, cannot be underestimated in the context of a reflexology treatment.

'The greatest sense in our body is our touch sense. It is probably the chief sense in the processes of sleeping and waking; it gives us our knowledge of depth or thickness and form; we feel, we love and hate, are touchy and are touched, through the touch corpuscles of our skin.'

J. Lionel Taylor, 1921

When we are born, touch is our most heightened sense, it is our first form of communication, being beyond words. Bertrand Russell said '... our whole conception of what exists outside us, is based on the sense of touch'. To be cared for and touched is a basic human need and vital for the development of each individual. Ashley Montagu in his book 'Touching' says,

'By being stroked and caressed, and carried, and cuddled, comforted, and cooed to, by being loved, the child learns to stroke and caress and cuddle, comfort and coo, and to love others.'

Tiffany Field, at the Touch Research Institute in Miami, has conducted extensive studies into the value of touch, in particular for premature babies.These studies show how, with regular massage, premature babies had a greater weight gain than babies who were not massaged. Perhaps, more importantly, this improvement in development had continued when the babies reached one year old.

In Sweden, the Axelsons Gymnastiska Institut has conducted studies with children. After integrating massage into the daily routine in more than one thousand kindergartens, the children became calmer, could concentrate more easily and were more sociable in groups.

Touching is not a part of daily life in Western cultures and is often associated with inhibitions and even taboos in certain situations. With reflexology, clients can receive a 'safe' and appropriate touch which, in itself, can have a beneficially therapeutic effect.

The skin can often reflect emotions, for example we blush with embarassment. Tension and stress can present themselves in the form of skin conditions such as eczema and psoriasis. Often the words that someone uses to describe their skin also matches their emotional state, for example someone who is frustrated and restricted may say that their skin is 'breaking out', as though that is the only breaking out that they are capable of.

The reflex areas for the sensory organs and associated areas are shown in *Figure 12.1.*

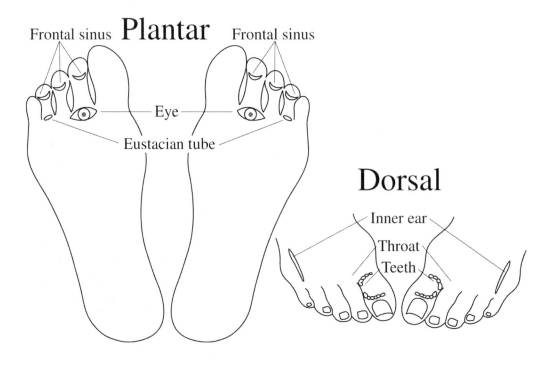

Figure 12.1

Case studies

1. Client details — Emma. Age 42. Married with no children. Senior clerical officer. There have been redundancies at work and, while her own job appears to be secure, she now has an increased workload with fewer staff.

Presenting symptoms: Chronic tinnitus. She has had this problem for ten years, it is aggravated by stress and at present it is very evident and constant. She is inevitably depressed because of this. She finds it difficult to concentrate and is exhausted, both physically and mentally.

She is very familiar with this long term condition and has realistic expectations of the treatment outcome. She would like to achieve a reduction in the symptoms so that it feels manageable to her again. She is very aware of the effect of stress on the tinnitus and on her generally.

Treatment: On presentation the pituitary, forebrain and neck reflexes are all tender and tense. Relevant links are used, ie. forebrain to base of spine, pituitary to adrenal and neck to jaw. The inner ear reflexes are extremely sensitive, especially on the left foot. These are worked lightly and returned to several times during a treatment. The practitioner has shown Emma the inner ear reflexes on the hands and she works these, herself, gently each day between the sessions. She finds this helpful and can monitor the condition by the degree of sensitivity.

Immediately after each treatment the ear noises are louder for two days and then become much quieter for varying lengths of time; sometimes this lasts for one week and sometimes for as long as two weeks, the length of improvement reflecting her stress levels.

After the third treatment, Emma began to relax during the session. She enjoys this now, looks forward to it and feels that it helps her to cope with the stresses of her job better than before. The neck and jaw area is always very tender and she now realises exactly how much tension she can hold there; often she can be so tense that when she wakes up her jaw is clenched. The reflexology has made her aware of this, so she practises some simple relaxation techniques that seem to be helping before going to sleep .

2. Client details — Elsie. Age 54. Married. One adult daughter. She is very self-conscious, timid and frequently apologises for herself for no apparent reason. She is a secretary.

Presenting symptom: High blood pressure. She says that this frightens her. She talks a lot and, again, apologises for this, saying that she is nervous. Often in this conversation she talks about situations in her life when she has missed opportunities because she was afraid to take a risk, and she seems to be generally fearful.

Treatment: At the first treatment she was nervous and anxious. This was mainly a foot massage session with lots of reassurance. She was obviously unhappy with her working situation and described her job as 'the general skivvy'; she feels that she is given work that no-one else will do. However, she also feels that this is her own fault because she doesn't speak up for herself and just accepts what is given to her. Her feet were extremely tense. As treatment progressed she relaxed and more reflexology could be used. The neck and shoulder reflexes are always tight and tender initially but they do now relax during the treatment. The thyroid link is very powerful and feels slightly uncomfortable for her. Also the throat reflex area is tender and she has frequent throat infections. It is as though this emphasises her inability to communicate and she, herself, says that she finds it difficult to express herself.

Over a period of six months she changed in appearance, looking more confident and smiling more often. She has quietly become more confident at work, being able to tell her immediate superior how she feels — she feels happier there now. She still has the same apologetic manner but does relax and enjoy the sessions more. For relaxation, and to help her feel more empowered, she was guided through a basic breathing and relaxation exercise. She still finds it difficult to be assertive at work but now, instead of bottling her feelings up, she practises this relaxation sequence at her desk. Her blood pressure has gone down very slightly and she is less anxious about it. She also has fewer throat infections.

References

Axelsons Gymnastiska Institut, Box 6475,11382 Stockholm

Montagu A (1986) *Touching*. Harper and Row, USA: 126

Taylor JL (1921) The Stages of Human Life. In: Montagu A (1986) *Touching*. Harper and Row, New York: 3

Touch Research Institute,University of Miami, School of Medicine, PO Box 016820, Miami, FL33101, USA

General points to remember about the 'linking' technique:

- The responses are a reflection of the subtle energy levels of each client and, as such, they won't necessarily be obvious and vibrant. They differ from person to person and from treatment to treatment, the ideal situation being for the energy to match the nature of the person. The application is a non-judgemental acceptance of how that person is functioning at that time.

- Whatever is felt, is a true and correct feeling operating on an instinctive level, and is beyond words.

- It is not necessary, in fact probably not advisable, to work all the 'links' within each session, but instead to be selective, using ones that are appropriate.

- Generally speaking, the stronger the reaction then the more effective the 'link' will be.

- If practical, hold the link until the response fades away.

- Trust the intuitive response.

13
Precision reflexology procedure and charts

'Linking' is one technique, forming part of a full reflexology treatment. The precision reflexology chart (see *Figure 13.1*) is used as a 'map' to cover the whole of the body.

Hand treatments can also be used, see *Figure 13.2*. Hand reflexology can be given if the feet are inaccessible for one reason or another, for instance in cases of severe injury or infection. Occasionally it is a client's preference. Working on hands is an invaluable form of reinforcement between sessions and a genuine way to establish the principle of self-help.

The main stroke used within treatments is a slow rotating thumb pressure, interspersed with effleurage and percussion massage strokes. It is always beneficial to commence a treatment with a general foot massage sequence (including mobilisation of the foot and ankle) so as to reassure the client, to give him/her time to settle down, to introduce an element of relaxation and for the practitioner to begin to assess the level of stress within each person.

The overall procedure is outlined in the chart shown in *Figure 13.3* with 'links' being integrated in the relevant areas. This is obviously a standard, general treatment which would be adapted to suit each individual, with more or less emphasis on certain areas. The practitioner is guided by the sensitivity in his/her hands, by intuition, by the client's responses and by an holistic knowledge of the anatomy and physiology of the body.

As with all massage, there are a variety of strokes and styles that can be adapted, the overall principle being that the client should feel at times interested, curious, involved, or relaxed but always secure, with a sense of being held safely.

Generally, the deeper the stroke, the more effective it will be. Tenderness usually indicates an imbalance so the pressure used should always be within comfortable limits. If clients receiving a treatment are constantly fearful and anticipating pain then they cannot, consciously or unconsciously, allow themselves to heal. The aim is for the body to be in a relaxed, parasympathetic state. On tender areas it is more effective to apply comfortable pressure and then to return to the same reflex several times during the treatment (and in subsequent ones), each time being able to use slightly more pressure. In this way, the body can heal in its own time gradually and effectively, without force. The 'linking' technique is especially helpful on tender reflexes because the treatment can be energetic with a very light touch.

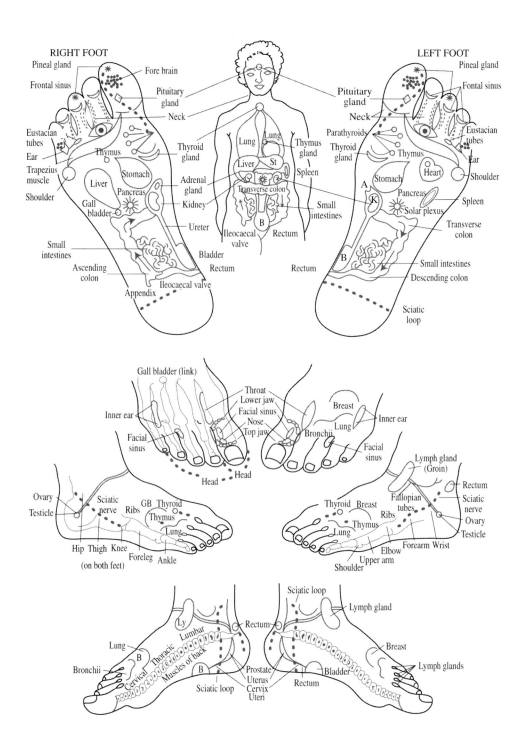

Figure 13.1: Precision reflexology chart

Hand chart

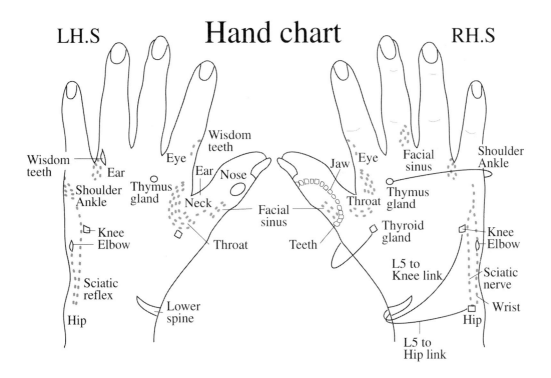

LH.S

RH.S

Wisdom teeth

Eye

Wisdom teeth

Ear

Nose

Jaw

Eye

Facial sinus

Shoulder Ankle

Wisdom teeth

Ear

Thymus gland

Neck

Throat

Thymus gland

Shoulder Ankle

Facial sinus

Thyroid gland

Knee Elbow

Knee Elbow

Throat

Teeth

Sciatic nerve

Sciatic reflex

L5 to Knee link

Wrist

Hip

Lower spine

Hip

L5 to Hip link

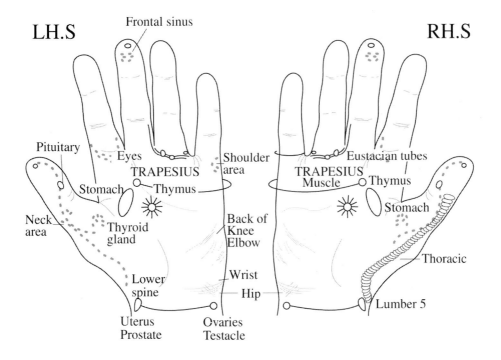

LH.S

Frontal sinus

RH.S

Pituitary

Eyes

TRAPESIUS

Shoulder area

Eustacian tubes

TRAPESIUS Muscle

Thymus

Stomach

Thymus

Stomach

Neck area

Thyroid gland

Back of Knee Elbow

Thoracic

Lower spine

Wrist

Hip

Lumber 5

Uterus Prostate

Ovaries Testacle

Figure 13.2

Figure 13.3: Precision reflexology procedure

NB: 'L' indicates where a link can be used if appropriate

Relaxation massage — both feet

Right foot:	*Left foot:*
Solar plexus	Solar plexus
Thyroid gland L	Thyroid gland L
Parathyroid glands L	Parathyroid glands L
Neck L	Neck L
Pituitary gland	Pituitary gland
Forebrain L	Forebrain L
Pineal gland L	Pineal gland L
Sinuses	Sinuses
Throat	Throat
Eyes	Eyes
Eustachian tubes	Eustachian tubes
Ears	Ears
Bronchi	Bronchi
Lungs — dorsal and plantar aspect of foot L	Lungs — dorsal and plantar aspect of foot L
Lymph area — dorsal	Lymph area — dorsal
Breast	Breast
Shoulders L	Shoulders L
Thymus L	Thymus L
Diaphragm	Diaphragm
Liver	Heart
Gall bladder L	Stomach
Stomach	Spleen
Small intestines	Pancreas
Ascending colon	Small intestines
First half of transverse colon	Second half of transverse colon
Kidney	Descending colon
Adrenal gland L	Sigmoid colon to rectum
Ureter to bladder	Kidney
Muscles of spine	Adrenal gland L
Spine L	Ureter to bladder
Leg L	Muscles of spine
Arm L	Spine L
Reproductive system L	Leg L
Lymph — back of heel	Arm L
Effleurage	Reproductive system L
	Lymph — back of heel
	Effleurage

Finishing with a reassuring hold of both feet to accompany the client's deep breathing

A parallel principle here is the Chinese one of saying that the quickest way from A to B is not in a direct line (see *Figure 13.4)* as this can be too forceful, being met with resistance and, thus, rejected. But rather, to take a softer approach (see *Figure 13.5*) which can be readily accepted. There is also a Yogic theme which maintains that it is possible to be strong and relaxed **at the same time**. This says that control and tension are not synonymous. It is possible to achieve a state of balance with both steadiness (in Sanskrit this is Stkira) and relaxation (Sukha) present together. Similarities with this Yogic philosophy and the application of reflexology can be seen in the use of a firm and gentle touch.

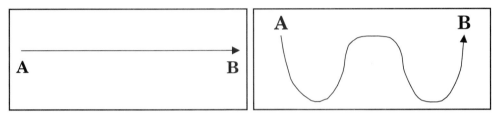

Figure 13.4

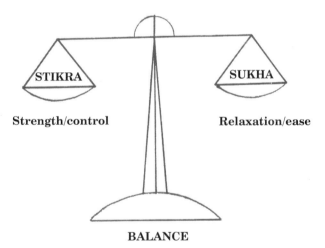

Figure 13.5

If we accept that the feet represent the energy of the body, then each reflex area needs to be handled in an appropriate way. Firmer pressure can be applied to the more robust areas, eg. the shoulders, and a lighter touch to the more delicate structures, eg. the eyes. Also, receiving the treatment will feel different for different points, eg. the intestines tend to produce dull, bruised reactions, with the neurological areas being sharp and tingling.

There is an endless variety of reactions that can be felt by the practitioner. For instance, the reflexes can feel crystalline, bubbly, fibrous, hot, cold, soft or tense. Also there are less tangible responses which have been described using words such as energetic, lethargic, sharp, dull, empty and full. The sensitive practitioner can decipher this information, and relate it to the particular organ, and to the nature of each client, in order to establish if it is appropriate or not.

Client reactions differ, some isolating response purely to the feet, with others having sensations in the related body part. Both are equally valid — reflecting how that person is functioning at that time.

Improvements in health are rarely steady and consistent but usually progress with natural fluctuations, reflecting the 'ups and downs' that clients report. Thankfully, this sequence of events often results in the benefits being sustained. The power of the healing needs to be in the client's own time and own way and not as a result of the will or ego of the practitioner.

The consultation situation aims to be, at times, pleasurable and relaxing and, at other times, challenging and provocative, while always being constructive and positive.

By holding the solar plexus reflex point at the beginning of the treatment, it is possible to have a tangible sense of the client's true nature. The pressure used needs to feel positive and acceptable, but not painful. This varies from person to person and from treatment to treatment. Often the reality is quite different from the presentation of the person; this reflex point may feel sensitive and vulnerable or, indeed, robust and energetic, either state often indicating a quite different persona from the one that the client presents.

The pressure used is matched to the health, sensitivity, and nature of each part of the body. For example, no caring person would apply strong pressure to the top of someone's head, therefore light touch is applied to the top of each toe. In the same way, the reflexology pressure used on the large muscles of the shoulders will differ considerably from that used on delicate structures such as the sinuses. Likewise, a healthy liver is a robust organ so a deep pressure can be applied whereas, on the more fragile kidneys, a lighter touch would be equally effective.

Contraindications

There are few times when reflexology would not be recommended but, as each treatment is adapted to the individual recipient, there may be situations when caution is needed. General, overall guidelines, include:

- Conditions such as deep vein thrombosis or phlebitis, which would not respond favourably to stimulation, should not be treated.
- Patients taking regular medication, such as thyroxin or insulin, should be made aware that reflexology can positively affect these conditions so that they need to monitor themselves in case they need to adjust their medication.
- During pregnancy it is advisable to avoid treatment for the first thirteen weeks until the pregnancy is established. Thereafter, as a precautionary measure, do not work the reproductive areas or the pituitary gland. Extreme caution is needed if the woman has a history of unstable pregnancies.
- Clients with heart conditions can be treated with the recommendation of their doctor. Obviously, the heart area itself is avoided. In these cases there is considerable stress so the relaxation achieved during a treatment has a positive effect.
- Cancer patients in general will benefit from the treatment. However, because of the effect on the immune system, it is advisable not to treat if they are receiving chemotherapy or radiotherapy. Obviously the reflex for the area where the cancer has occurred should be avoided. In terminal cases, the positive effect of touch and tender loving care cannot be underestimated.

These are general guidelines and each situation must be considered in its own right. An important principle is that the practitioner and the client/patient must both feel confident to proceed with the treatment.

14
Complete holistic healthcare

Complementary health practitioners share an overriding ethos within their work, and this has two major aims:

- to restore a state of homeostasis to the health of each client
- to encourage each client to begin to take responsibility for his/her own health.

Each therapy uses its own particular approach to try to achieve these aims but also, in order to maintain the benefits over a period of time, it is essential to consider how each individual can look after him/herself. Surely what really matters is what happens between the consultations. The truly important aspect of each person's health status must surely be how he/she can restore, and realistically maintain, health and well-being. Each person should be able to do this in varying degrees dependent upon their age, lifestyle and overall state of health. Obviously reflexologists use their own techniques to achieve this situation but we cannot underestimate the value of self-care; the ultimate power is in the hands of the client/patient. The self-esteem resulting from this empowerment has, in turn, a positive effect on health (see *Figure 14.1*).

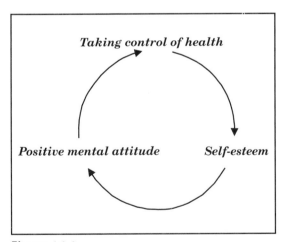

Figure 14.1

The consultation often acts as a catalyst to 'trigger' motivation for the client to act. Hopefully, as clients begin to ask themselves 'how am I today?' and 'how do I feel?', the next question will be 'what can I do about it?'. Each person needs strategies or life-skills to apply to this increased self-awareness. Ideally, any changes need to be manageable, gradual and certainly not a cause of stress in themselves. The steps taken need to feel realistic; in this way they can become an acceptable and enjoyable part of life.

Ways of achieving self-care

Diet and nutrition: the aim being to receive energy from food and to eat with enjoyment in a relaxed, sociable manner. The guidelines for each person need to be feasible, even if challenging as any sense of resentment or denial can cause an imbalance and tension in itself. The most appropriate dictum is to aim for food that has been treated as little as possible and that is as fresh as possible. Modern food production, with techniques such as genetic engineering and the extensive use of pesticides, presents obstacles to be overcome.The intake of 'non-foods' such as sugar and salt, and stimulants such as coffee, alcohol and nicotine should be avoided or, at least, reduced. There may be specific advice for some health problems, for instance to reduce acid-forming foods in cases of arthritis, to reduce dairy foods for some respiratory problems or to increase the intake of fresh, organic fruit and vegetables in order to boost immunity.

There is always an emotional element with food; how and what we eat is the ultimate expression of our self-care. The reflexology consultation can perhaps begin to address these issues as the client/practitoner relationship develops.

Exercise: energy is movement. Obviously this needs to be matched to the ability, lifestyle and temperament of each person. An equal sense of achievement can be obtained for one person by completing a six-mile run and, for another, by walking to the garden gate. Again the principle should be one of enjoyment. This may be a specific exercise for a particular problem, for instance to reduce congestion and pain during menstruation, or a routine for general fitness. The sense of well-being achieved by regular exercise has a positive effect on all levels; the physical benefits are obvious, stress is reduced and the spirits are restored by the release of the natural relaxator, the endorphins.

Relaxation: to achieve some exclusive time for oneself breaks the stress response and has a positive effect physically, mentally and spiritually. This may be of a certain design, for example, Yoga or Tai Chi; or it may be by creating a few quiet moments within the day, such as by going for a walk in the country. Being surrounded by beautiful countryside, feeling a part of nature, reaffirms the Oriental belief that each human spirit is a part of the wider universe.

The body is designed to cope with short-term stress; damage occurs if this becomes constant and long-term. This situation depletes the body's energy whether it be physical, emotional or spiritual. Relaxation with conscious awareness not only prevents the accumulation of stress, but also increases self-awareness of how it feels to be relaxed in constrast to how it feels to be stressed. Often stress has gradually built-up over a period of time and relaxation provides a way of standing back to review the situation. Stress can be seen as a response to change, accompanied by a feeling of loss of control — involvement with one's own healthcare can help to counter these feelings. Energy levels can be restored so that, with increased vitality and clarity of mind, the individual can function in a more efficient and self-contained manner. Leonardo da Vinci said,

> '*Every now and then go away, have a little relaxation, for when you come back to your work your judgement will be surer; since to remain constantly at work will cause you to lose power of judgement. Go some distance away because the work appears smaller and more of it can be taken in at a glance, and a lack of harmony or proportion is more readily seen.*'

Does the last sentence refer to life or art, or both? Often success and stress are thought to be synonomous with each other. The Yogic principle mentioned in *Chapter 13* demonstrates that strength and control (stkira) can exist side-by-side with relaxation and ease (sukha), in fact the one should be balanced with the other. Complementary therapy acknowledges the unique nature of each individual, this is evident in the approach to stress; what is stressful to one person is simply healthy motivation to another. Equally, what may seem like trivial situations to one person, to another present major opportunities for stress and tension. Within a consultation each individual response is obviously respected as being how that individual functions. Just as unique is the manner of relaxation; some prefer a set, focused procedure with specific breathing techniques, while others achieve the same benefits by consciously creating some 'time out'.

> '*You cannot lead a balanced life without periods of relaxation. This is not the same as sleep, which is a combination of restfulness and specific internal activity. Relaxation is the vital process of letting-go.*'

Howard Kent, 1993

Relaxation may sound gentle and soft, and this is so, but it can have a powerful effect.

Breathing: many people have become lazy in their manner of breathing. Often, simple, deep breathing techniques can have a dramatic effect on energy levels. Deep breathing is simple and totally non-invasive. No special equipment is needed, neither is any external intervention. It acts as an internal massage, has a beneficial effect on every system of the body and restores a sense of calm. Specific breathing techniques can be matched to each individual and each situation. It may be appropriate to adopt slow, deep breathing to reduce tension and to help regain control in stressful situations or to practice energising breaths to counter tiredness. It can take quite a time to relinquish established patterns of breathing and to re-learn new ones.

Breathing is taken for granted but all stresses and strains will affect the flow of breath, so we can never afford to ignore it. Huge benefits are to be gained from being aware of the movement and value of each breath. A strong sense of self-control and self-management, that is both simple and powerful, can be achieved by being in charge of this vital process.

We can affect how we feel and function with how we breathe. In stressful situations, the vital instinctive response for the body is to breathe rapidly. The effect of slow, deep breathing is to reverse the stress response by sending calming messages around the body and mind to say that it is not a stressful situation. Specific visualisation methods, in conjunction with breathing patterns, can be used to help alleviate tension and pain.

> *'Breathe naturally, without forcing. No pressure, no disturbance, nothing should interfere with the simple, tide-like movement of our lungs as we breathe in and out.'*

Vanda Scaravelli, 1991

Each of these aspects can be introduced into the consultation as, and when, the practitioner feels appropriate — the skill being to know how much to introduce and when? This is a measure of the quality of each therapeutic relationship — so that clients feel empowered as well as secure and supported.

Holistic foot care

Reflexologists believe that any imbalances within the system are reflected in the feet so it seems reasonable to believe that any problems with the feet themselves could be reflected in the body. It would also seem fair to accept that this is a two-way connection. Therefore, a valuable form of self-help is to take good care of our feet. The most obvious and effective way of doing this is in the selection of the shoes that we put on.

Badly fitting shoes cause foot problems, such as bunions and corns (that can have an effect in reflexology terms on the rest of the body), and impact on the structure of the body, especially the spine, by interfering with natural balance and alignment.

Someone's body only needs to be slightly out of line, for instance they may stand with more weight on one foot than on the other, and this, over the years, can result in chronic back pain as all the structures of the body try to compensate. This can sometimes be corrected by being aware of the misalignment and by adjusting posture, or by exercises to strengthen the weaker area.

Often skeletal problems, particularly of the spine, pelvis and ankles can be alleviated by professional advice on foot mechanics. Such advice can provide support, reduce discomfort and also help to re-align the structures of the body. An example of this is a thirty-five year old woman who presented with acute lumbar spine pain. She received reflexology which gave her short-term relief but, to provide long-term care, it was necessary to address the cause of the problem. She had always been knock-kneed and when she walked she swung her legs slightly out to the side with each step. She was referred to a local shoe-maker who also practised foot mechanics — he made her some shoes with specifically designed supports in the sole and the result was dramatic. Within weeks, her back problem had vanished and she could walk for long distances which had previously been impossible.

Shoes which are made to measure for each individual, not only match the feet, but also match the person and their unique body dynamics.

References

Kent H (1993) *The Complete Yoga Course*. Headline Book Publishing Ltd, London: 31

Scaravelli V (1991) *Awakening the Spine*. Harper Collins Publishers, London: 176

15
Precision reflexology — a complementary therapy

The primary focus behind all complementary therapy is to **care** rather than to **cure**. Reflexology provides an opportunity for people to be cared for and, more importantly, to begin to care for themselves. It gives exclusive time which is valuable and healing in itself.

There is no one defined way to be well or unwell and the symptoms that people describe are their own way of saying that they are not well. Ideally, within the treatments, individuals can feel involved in their own healthcare and become aware of all the various aspects of life that contribute to their state of health. This sense of empowerment may be apparent in practical ways, represented by realistic and appropriate life-style changes. The effect of this 'self-help' approach increases self-esteem, resulting in an increased sense of well-being. There may be less obvious changes as this involvement also provokes questions such as 'why this problem and why at this time?' or 'how does this make me feel?' with rather less attention to the original symptom. The answers to questions like these can demonstrate how the body **is** the emotions. The conscious realisation of this fact can then influence future healthcare. Sometimes, the emotional connection is easy to see, but sometimes it is not such an obvious attachment. It is important not to involve any sense of blame or guilt in this process. More total understanding of the deeper meaning behind an illness allows an individual to take responsibility for his/her healthcare on all levels of being.

The actual phrase 'to take responsibility for one's own healthcare' sounds challenging and positive but it can seem overwhelming and daunting. Individuals will, quite rightly, approach this prospect to varying degrees and in various ways, some with great enthusiasm and some tentatively. The manner adopted will reflect an individual's attitude of mind, overall state of health and background: each client bringing his/her own agenda to a consultation. Ideally, the process can be constructive and worthwhile, bringing an understanding of how we feel when we are well or unwell. Reflexology consultations, along with other complementary therapies, create a situation where people can become more fully acquainted with themselves.

The ultimate aim is for each person to be aware that, whether they are well or unwell, the whole experience of treatment can be rewarding. If they have a problem, it is not something alien that needs to be got rid of but, rather, it is an integral part of them and, as such, it is something to be understood and accepted. It is not a case of fighting or of being defeated but of accepting while maintaining a strong sense of self and moving forward positively. Also, the state of health at that time is not an isolated incident but part of an ongoing process.

This idea of understanding symptoms, almost of forming a relationship with them, may seem impossible but it can be paralled to the parent/child relationship that can seem equally impossible. At times this can be harmonious and easy and, at other times, it can be challenging and provocative. For any relationship to be worthwhile, it should be dynamic and constantly changing — situations arise that could be potentially confrontational. A child can be controlled and suppressed, providing acceptable and immediate order but also creating a distance between the parent and the child, or attention can be given to the child's nature, attempting to understand how the situation arose. This latter approach requires more time and energy and is less conventional. However, ultimately it is the more rewarding for all concerned, and certainly the relationship that develops as a result is deeper, stronger and richer and will continue to grow and flourish.

The various elements within precision reflexology treatments, the practitioner's skill and intuitive sense, the client's involvement and the relationship between the client and the practitioner, all support the process of understanding and growth.

'If you ask for kindness, be kind
If you ask for truth, be true
What you give of yourself, you find
This world is a reflex of you.'

Gandhi

Recommended reading

Blythman J (1996) *The Food We Eat*. Michael Joseph, London

Colburn T, Myers JP, Dumanoski D (1996) *Stolen Future*. Little, Brown and Company, USA

Cormack M, Mitchell A (1998) *The Therapeutic Relationship in Complementary Health Care*. Churchill Livingstone, Edinburgh

Issel C (1990) *Reflexology, Art, Science and History*. New Frontier, Sacramento, California

Mitchell S (1998) *Naturopathy*. ElementBooks, Shaftesbury

Montagu A (1986) *Touching*. Harper and Row, USA

Pert CB (1998) *Molecules of Emotion* . Simon and Schuster, USA

The Sivananda Yoga Centre (Lidell, Rabinovitch and Rabinovitch). (1983) *The Book of Yoga*. Ebury Press, London

Walker K (1996) *Hand Reflexology*. Quay Books, Salisbury

Useful addresses

Federation of Precision Reflexology
The School of Complementary Health
38 South Street
Exeter EX1 1ED

Association of Reflexologists
27 Old Gloucester Street
London WC1N 3XX

Chuckle Shoes
3 Newbridge Street
Exeter

Prue Miskin
2 Devon House Drive
Bovey Tracey
Devon

Index